The A to

T0329492

Introduction

While writing the A to Z of ~~...~~
apparent that a full discuss ~~...~~
along with the inclusion of the Thyroid gland, for which there had been many
requests. Due to the complexity of hormonal interactions and their overlapping
effects, flow charts, tables and abbreviations are used extensively in this book.
"New" hormones are being discovered all the time, or "old" ones are being
renamed, hence there is extensive cross referencing of hormone names.

The immune system and its detailed interactions needs an A to Z book of
its own, so although discussed in this book, this subject will be dealt with
extensively in *The A To Z of the Immune.System*, in which the spectrum of
autoimmune diseases, the detailed role of the thymus and the lymphatic system
will also be closely examined.

The A to Zs may be viewed on 2 sites –
www.amandasatoz.com and
http://www.aspenpharma.com.au/atlas/student.htm
Feedback may be left at
anatomy.update@gmail.com / **medicalamanda@gmail.com**
and it is always appreciated.

Acknowledgement

Thank you Aspenpharmacare Australia particularly Greg Lan, Rob Koster,
Richard Clement and Peter Penn, for your support and assistance. This is
the 10th year of the A to Zs which continue to expand and now consist of 15
books, and other associated projects. They fill a need in the medical and
health community, and cover the basic anatomical concepts in the normal and
increasingly in the abnormal. And they continue to grow - thank you.

Dedication

To one of my dearest friends and colleagues Rob Koster. Thank you.

How to use this book

The format of this A to Z book has been maintained. The ***Common Terms
of Endocrinology section*** contains brief summaries of terms & concepts
necessary for the understanding of the influences & formation of this system.
The Hormone & Other Substances section contains the **Hormone Table A
to Z** which lists all the major hormones of the endocrine system. This section
also includes other important influential substances e.g. the precursors of
Hormones, the structures and basic chemistry of their components, the Amino
acids & Cholesterol. It also includes the Vitamins.

The Organs & Tissues of Endocrinology section contains **the Endocrine Organs and their Hormones Table** which lists all the major Organs and the hormones they secrete. Additional information relating to these tables can be found in their respective sections in the A to Z format.

The section on *Pathways & Processes* summarizes the major hormone pathways and interactions

So as usual *think of it and then find it* is the motto of *the A to Zs* and continues to be the structure behind the books.

Thank you
A. L. Neill
BSc MSc MBBS PhD FACBS

ISBN 978-1-921930-07-2

9 781921 930072

TABLE OF CONTENTS

HORMONES & OTHER SUBSTANCES

HORMONE TABLE - A TO Z

ORGANS & TISSUES OF ENDOCRINOLOGY

PATHWAYS & PROCESSES

Abbreviations of the terms used in Endocrinology

5HT	5-hydroxytryptamine, serotonin

A

a	artery
aa	anastomosis (ses)
AA	amino acid
AAAH	**aromatic amino-acid hydroxylase**
AADC	**aromatic L-amino acid decarboxylase**
Ab	antibody
AB	antibiotic
ABC	ATP-binding cassette family of proteins
ABP	androgen binding protein
ACAT	**acetyl-CoA: cholesterol acetyltransferase** - permitting acetyl-CoA into the mitochondria
ACAT1	**acetyl-CoA acetyltransferase 1; acetoacetyl-CoA thiolase**, mitochondrial; involved in ketone body synthesis
ACAT2	**acetyl-CoA acetyltransferase 2; acetoacetyl-CoA thiolase**, cytoplasmic; involved in cholesterol biosynthesis
ACC2	**acetyl-CoA carboxylase**, expressed in heart, liver, skeletal muscle, mitochondrial targeting motif, found associated with CPT I
ACE	angiotensin converting enzyme
ACh	acetylcholine
AChR	acetylcholine receptor
ACOX1,2,3	peroxisomal fatty acyl-CoA oxidase 1, 2, & 3
ACP	acyl-carrier protein
ACTH	adrenocorticotrophic hormone / adrenal cortical H
ACS	**acyl-CoA synthetase**
ADH	antidiuretic hormone
ADP	adenosine diphosphate
Ag	antigen
AGL	glycogen debranching enzyme, GDE
AgRP	agouti-related peptide, hypothalamic neuropeptide antagonizes α-MSH
AI	adequate intake - referring to vitamins etc
AI	autoimmune
AID	autoimmune diseases / disorder
AIS	androgen insensitivity syndrome
AITD	autoimmune thyroid disease

AKA	also known as
alt	alternative
ALT	**alanine transaminase AKA serum glutamate pyruvate transaminase**
ALXR	lipoxin receptor
AMP	adenosine monophophate
AMPK	**AMP-activated protein kinase**
ANP	atrial natriuretic peptide AKA atrial natriuretic factor ANF
ANS	autonomic nervous system
ant.	anterior
anti-If	anti-inflammatory
AP	action potential
APC	activated protein C
AR	androgen receptor
ARC	arcuate nucleus, region of the hypothalamus involved in feeding behaviour
art.	artery
AS	alternative spelling
ASP	acylation stimulating protein
AT	adipose tissue
ATGL	**adipose triglyceride lipase**
ATL	aspirin-triggered lipoxin
ATP	adenosine triphosphate, major biological E source

B

b	bone
B	blood
BAT	brown adipose tissue
BBB	blood brain barrier
bc	because
BCAA	branched-chain amino acid
BCKD	**branched-chain α-ketoacid dehydrogenase**
BF	blood flow
BGLAP	osteocalcin AKA bone-γ-carboxyglutamic-acid-containing-protein
BM	basement membrane / bone marrow
b/n	between
BMP	bone morphogenetic protein
BMR	basal metabolic rate
BNP	brain natriuretic peptide
BP	blood pressure

BS	blood supply
BUN	blood urea nitrogen
BV	blood vessel

C

C	carbon
Ca / Ca^{2+}	calcium / calcium ion
CaCM	calcium calmodulin
CAH	congenital adrenal hyperplasia
cAMP	cyclic AMP
CAR	constitutive androstane receptor
CART	cocaine & amphetamine-regulated transcript; hypothalamic neuropeptide involved in feeding behaviour
CC	cerebral cortex
CCF	congestive cardiac failure / congestive heart failure
CCK	cholecystekinin
cdc	cell division cycle
CD	collecting ducts of the Ky
CDK	**cyclin-dependent kinase**
CEN	centromere
c.f.	as in / as demonstrated here
cGMP	cyclic GMP
CGRP	calcitonin gene related peptide
ChE	**cholinesterase**
CHO	carbohydrate
CK	**creatine kinase**
CL	corpus luteum
CLA	conjugated linoleic acid - ω-3 FA, purported to be helpful against obesity & DM2
cm	cell membrane
CNS	central nervous system
COC	combined oral contraceptives (i.e. oestrogens + progesterones)
COMT	**catecholamine-O-methyltransferase**
CORT	cortistatin
CoQ	coenzyme Q; ubiquinone
COX	**cyclo oxygenase; COX1 & COX2**
CP	creatinine phosphate
CPK or CK	**creatine phopshokinase: creatine kinase**
CRBP	cellular retinol binding protein
CREB	cAMP response element-binding protein
CRF	corticotropin-releasing factor (hormone)

CSF	colony stimulating factor / cerebrospinal fluid
CT	connective tissue
CVA	cerebrovascular accident AKA stroke
CVD	cardiovascular disease
CVS	cardiovascular system
CYP	nomenclature prefix for cytochrome P450 class of enzymes
CYP7A1	**cholesterol 7-hydroxylase**; rate-limiting enzyme of classic pathway for bile acid synthesis
CYP8B1	**sterol 12α-hydroxylase**; bile acid synthesizing enzyme
CYP11A1	**P450 side-chain cleavage enzyme**, AKA **desmolase** AKA **cholesterol desmolase, 20,22 desmolase**; involved in steroid H synthesis
CYP11B1	**11β-hydroxylase**, AKA **P450c11**; involved in steroid H synthesis
CYP11B2	**aldosterone synthase**, AKA **18α-hydroxylase** or **P450c18**; involved in adrenal steroid hormone synthesis
CYP17A1	has 2 activities: **17α-hydroxylase & 17,20-lyase**, AKA **P450c17**; involved in steroid H synthesis
CYP19A1	**aromatase**, AKA **oestrogen synthetase**; involved in steroid H synthesis
CYP21A2	**21-hydroxylase**; involved in steroid H synthesis; AKA **CYP21 & CYP21B**

D

DCT	distal convoluted tubules (of the Ky)
DDx	differential diagnosis
DG	diglycerides
DHA	docasahexaenoic acid; important ω-3 FA
DHAP	dihydroxyacetone phosphate
DHEA	dehydroepiandosterone AKA androstenolone AKA prasterone
DHEA-S	dehydroepiandosterone sulphate
DHT	dihydrotestosterone
DKA	diabetic ketoacidosis
DLMO	dim light melatonin onset
DM	diabetes mellitus
DM1	Diabetes mellitus type 1 – insulin dependant
DM2	Diabeltes mellitus type 2 – non –insulin dependant
DMG	dimethyglycine
DMN	dorsomedial hypothalamic nucleus; involved in stimulating GIT activity
DNP	dinitrophenol; compound that uncouples e flow from ATP production
DOC	deoxy-corticosterone

Dol	dolichol
DOPA	3,4-dihydrophenylalanine
DSI	depolarization-induced suppression of inhibition; a term relating to neurochemical transmission in the CNS
DT	digestive tract

E

e	electron
E	energy
EC	extracellular
ECF	extracellular fluid
ECM	extracellular matrix
ECT	extracellular T
EFA	essential fatty acids
EGF	epidermal growth factor
eNOS	**endothelial nitric oxide synthase**
EOM	extra ocular muscles
EPA	eicosapentaenoic acid; important ω-3 FA, precursor for PGs & PGIs
EPI	extrinsic pathway inhibitor
EPO	erythropoietin
ER	endoplasmic reticulum

F

F6P	fructose -6-phosphate
FA	fatty acids
FAAH	**fatty acid amide hydrolase**
FABPc	cytosolic FA-binding protein
FAPα	fibroblast activation protein alpha
FAS	**fatty acid synthase**
FATP	fatty acid transport protein; six family members FATP1 – FATP6
FFA	free fatty acid
FGF	fibroblast growth factor
FGFR	fibroblast growth factor receptor
FH	familial hypercholesterolemia
FIZZ	found in inflammatory zone: a family of proteins that includes resistin AKA FIZZ3
FPG	fasting plasma glucose
FPP	farnesyl pyrophosphate
FSH	follicle-stimulating hormone

G

GA	golgi apparatus
G0S2	G_0/G_1 switch protein 2; peptide inhibitor of adipose TG lipase (ATGL) expressed by mononuclear cells
G1P	glucose-1-phosphate
G6P	glucose 6-phosphate
GABA	γ-amino butyric acid
GAD	**glutamic acid decarboxylase**
GAG	glycosaminoglycan
GAL	galanin
GALT	gut associated lymphoid tissue
GAP	GTPase activating protein
GB	gall bladder
Gb3	globotriaosylceramide; predominant glycolipid accumulating in Fabry disease, a lysosomal storage disease
GBD	glycogen-binding domain
GCC	glycine cleavage complex
GCG	glucogen
G-CSF	granulocyte colony stimulating factor
GD	Grave's disease
GDE	**glycogen debranching enzyme AKA amylo-1,6-glucosidase, AGL**
GEF	guanine nucleotide exchange factor
GF	growth factor
GFAT	**glutamine:fructose-6-phosphate aminotransferase 1**
GFR	glomerular filtration rate
GH	growth hormone AKA somatotropin
GIF	growth hormone-inhibiting factor AKA somatostatin AKA GIH growth hormone-inhibiting hormone (GHIH)
GIP	glucose-dependent insulinotropic peptide AKA gastric inhibitory peptide
GIT	gastrointestinal tract (stomach ➜ LI)
GlcNAc	*N*-acetylglucosamine
gld	gland
GLP-1, -2	glucagon-like peptide 1, -2
GLUT	glucose transporter (< 14 members) commonest GLUT1 ➜ GLUT5
GM	grey matter
GM-CSF	granulocyte-macrophage colony stimulating factor
GnRF	gonadotropin-releasing factor (hormone)
GPAT	**glycerol-3-phosphate acyltransferase**
GPCR	G-protein coupled receptor

GR	glucocorticoid receptor
GRACILE	growth retardation, aminoaciduria, cholestasis, iron overload, lactic acidosis, early death
GRF	growth hormone releasing factor AKA growth hormone releasing hormone (GRH) (also -GHRH / GHRF)
GS	**glycogen synthase AKA synthetase**
GSD	glycogen storage disease
GSH	glutathione
GSK	**glycogen synthase kinase**

H

H	hormone / hydrogen
HADH	**hydroxyacyl-CoA dehydrogenase/3-ketoacyl-CoA thiolase/ enoyl-CoA hydratase, subunit of the mito. trifunctional protein (MTP) that catalyses the last 3 steps of mito. FA β-oxidation**
hCG	human chorionic gonadotropin / trophin
HDL	high density lipoprotein
HF	hair follicle
HFCS	high fructose corn syrup
HGF	hepatocyte growth factor
HIOMT	**hydroxyindolo-O-methyltransferase**
HIV	human immunodeficiency virus
HMGR	**HMG-CoA reductase, 3-hydroxy-3-methylglutaryl-CoA reductase**
hPL	human placental lactogen
HR	heart rate
HRE	hormone response element
HRT	hormone replacement therapy
HSL	**hormone-sensitive lipase**
HT	hormone therapy
HTGL	**hepatic triglyceride lipase**

I

IAA	insulin auto-antibodies: anti-insulin antibodies
IAPP	amylin AKA islet amyloid polypeptide
IBABP	intestinal bile acid binding protein AKA FA-binding protein 6: FABP6
ic	intracellular
ICAM-1	intercellular cell adhesion molecule-1
ICCA	islet cell cytoplasmic antibodies
ICSA	islet cell surface antigen

IDDM	insulin-dependent diabetes mellitus AKA DM1
If	inflammation / inflammatory
IF	inhibiting factors
IFG	impaired fasting glucose
IFR	inflammatory response
IGF-1 -2	insulin-like growth factor 1 -2
IGFBP	insulin-like growth factor binding protein
IL	interleukin
IMR	immune response
In	infection
INF or IF	interferon: α-IFs are leukocyte-derived, β-IFs are fibroblast-derived, γ-IFs are lymphocyte derived
INS	insulin
IoL	islets of Langerhans
IR	insulin resistance
IU	international units
Iy	injury

J

JGA	juxtaglomerular apparatus of the kidney

K

KB	ketone body / ketones
Ky	kidney

L

L	left
LACI	lipoprotein-associated coagulation inhibitor
LAD	leukocyte adhesion deficiency
LAL	lysosomal acid lipase; important lysosomal enzyme involved in lipid metabolism; deficiency in LAL results in Wolman disease
LBP	L-bifunctional protein; involved in peroxisomal fatty acid β-oxidation
LCAD	long chain acylCoA dehydrogenase
LCAT	lecithin cholesterol acyltransferase
LCFA	long-chain fatty acid
LDL	low density lipoprotein
LDLR	low density lipoprotein receptor
LH	luteinizing hormone

LHRF	luteinizing hormone releasing factor
LI	large intestine
LN	lymph node
LNS	Lesch-Nyhan syndrome
LoH	loop of Henle (in the Ky)
LOX	**lipoxygenase; 3 members of enzyme family: LOX-5, LOX-12 & LOX-15**
LP	lamina propria
LPH	lipotrophin AKA lipotropin
L-PK	**liver isoform of pyruvate kinase**
LPL	**lipoprotein lipase**
LPL	lysophospholipid
LT	lymphoid tissue
LT	leukotriene
LX	lipoxin

M

MAO	**monoamine oxidase**
MCAD	**medium-chain acyl-CoA dehydrogenase**
MCD	**malonyl-CoA decarboxylase**
MCH	melanin concentrating hormone
MCP	monocyte chemotactic protein
M-CSF	macrophage colony stimulating factor
MD	macula densa cells of the kidney - distal part of the ascending limb of the LoH closely associated with the JGA
mem	membrane
MFS	Marfan syndrome
mØ	macrophage
MGL	**monoacylglyceride lipase**
MIP	mØ inhibitory protein
mm	mucous membranes
MMP	**matrix metalloproteinase**
mRNA	messenger ribonucleic acid
MPS	mucopolysaccharidosis; lysosomal storage diseases
MRt	metabolic rate
MR	mineralocorticoid receptor
mRNA	messenger RNA
MSH	melanocyte-stimulating hormone
MSUD	maple syrup urine disease
MTP	mitochondrial trifunctional protein; carries out the last three reactions of mitochondrial fatty acid β-oxidation
mu	muscle

| mv | microvilli |

N

N	nerve cell , neuron, nerve
NAD	normal / no abnormality
NADH	nicotinamide adenine dinucleotide
NADPH	nicotinamide adenine dinucleotide phosphate
NAT	serotonin-N-acteyl-transferase
N-CAM	neural cell adhesion molecule
NE	niacin equivalents
NEFA	non-esterified fatty acid
NGF	nerve growth factor
NGFR	nerve growth factor receptor
NHE	sodium hydrogen exchanger
NIDDM	non-insulin-dependent diabetes mellitus AKA DM2
nm	nuclear membrane
NO	nitric oxide
NOS	nitric oxide synthase: 3 types: nNOS (neuronal NOS, NOS-1) iNOS (inducible NOS, NOS-2), eNOS (endothelial NOS, NOS-3)
NPY	neuropeptide tyrosine
NS	nervous system / nerve supply
NSAID	non-steroidal anti-inflammatory drug
NT	neural tissue / nerve tissue
NTS	nucleus of the solitary tract (NTS for Lt. term *nucleus tractus solitarii*), specialized cells w/n the medulla responsible for sensations of taste & visceral sensations of stretch

O

OAA	oxaloacetic acid
OC	oral contraceptives
OD	overdose
OGTT	oral glucose tolerance test
OI	osteogenesis imperfecta
OP	osteoporosis
OPG	osteoprotegerin AKA osteoclastogenesis inhibitory factor
OPN	osteopontin
OSCP	oligomycin sensitivity-conferring protein; a protein that connect the F1 & F0 proteins of ATP synthase in the mitochondria
OTC	ornithine transcarbamoylase

P

P	phosphate
P450	**cytochrome P450 AKA CYP**
P450c11	proper nomenclature is **CYP11B1; 11β-hydroxylase**
P450c17	has 2 activities: **17α-hydroxylase & 17,20-lyase**; properly called **CYP17A1**
P450c18	proper nomenclature is **CYP11B2: aldosterone synthase, AKA 18α-hydroxylase**
P450c21	proper nomenclature is **CYP21A2: 21-hydroxylase**; AKA **CYP21** or **CYP21B**
P450ssc	proper nomenclature is **CYP11A1: P450 side-chain cleavage enzyme, AKA desmolase, cholesterol desmolase, & 20,22 desmolase**
PABA	4-aminobenzoic acid AKA para-aminobenzoic acid
PAF	platelet activating factor
PAI	plasminogen activator inhibitor; PAI-1, PAI-2
PaP	pancreatic polypeptide
PCOS	polycystic ovarian syndrome
PCR	polymerase chain reaction
PCT	proximal convoluted tubules (of the Ky)
PDGF	platelet-derived growth factor
PEP	phosphoenoylpyruvate
PEX	designation for peroxisomal proteins
PG	prostaglandin
PGD	prostoglandin D major prostoglandin produced by mast cells involved in asthma & other allergies
PGI	prostacyclin
PGK	**phosphoglycerate kinase**
PGS	**prostaglandin synthase; prostaglandin endoperoxide synthetase**
pl	isoelectric point
PIF	prolactin-release inhibiting factor (hormone)
PIH	prolactin inhibiting hormone AKA Dopamine
pit.	pituitary
PK	**pyruvate kinase**
PKA	**cAMP-dependent protein kinase**
PKC	**Ca^{2+}-phospholipid-dependent protein kinase**
PKD	**DNA-dependent protein kinase**
PKG	**cGMP-dependent protein kinase**
PKU	phenylketonuria
pl	plural
PLA_2	**phospholipase A_2**

PLP	pyridoxal phosphate
PMN	polymorphonuclear leukocyte
PMT	premenstral tension
PN	peripheral nerve
PNS	peripheral nervous system
PO	phosphate
post.	posterior
PP	polypeptide
PP	**protein phosphatase**
PPI	protein phosphatase inhibitor
PPP	pentose phosphate pathway
PGR	progesterone receptor
PPT	postpartum thyroiditis
PRF	prolactin-releasing factor
pro-If pro-IF	pro-inflammatory
prot.	protein
PRL	prolactin
PTH	parathyroid hormone
PTK	**protein tyrosine kinase**
PTP	**protein tyrosine phosphatase**
PUFA	polyunsaturated fatty acid
PVN	paraventricular nucleus, hypothalamic region involved in Oxytocin & ADH release
PVR	peripheral vascular resistance
PWS	Prader-Willi syndrome
PYY	peptide tyrosine tyrosine

R

R	right / amino acid side chain
R5P	ribose-5-phosphate
RANK	osteoclast surface receptor - binds to RANKL
RAAS	renin-angiotensin-aldosterone-system
RANKL	receptor activator of nuclear factor-kappaB ligand
RAR	retinoic acid receptor
RBC	red blood cell
RBM	red bone marrow / haemopoieitic (blood forming) bone marrow
RBP	retinol binding protein
RDS	respiratory distress syndrome
RDA	recommended dietary intake AKA recommended daily allowance
RER	rough endoplasmic reticulum

RF	releasing factors / releasing hormone
RIA	radioimmunoassay
RLN	relaxin
RNA	ribonucleic acid
ROS	reactive oxidative species AKA free radicals
rRNA	ribosomal RNA
RT	**reverse transcription, reverse transcriptase**
RTK	**receptor tyrosine kinase**
RXR	retinoid X receptor

S

SAA	serum amyloid A
SA	sexual activity
SCAD	**short chain acylCoA dehydrogenase**
SCN	suprachiasmatic nuclei
SE	side effects
SER	smooth endoplasmic reticulum
SGLT2	sodium-glucose co-transporter: target for treatment of hyperglycaemia in diabetes
SGOT	**serum glutamate oxalate transaminase**
SGPT	**serum glutamate pyruvate transaminase**
SHBG	sex hormone binding globulin
SI	small intestine
SIF	somatostatin, = GIF
sing	singular
SKM	skeletal muscle / striated muscle
SLE	systemic lupus erythematosis
SM	smooth muscle
SMRT	silencing mediator of retinoid & thyroid H receptor
SNS	sympathetic nervous system
SR	sarcoplasmic reticulum
SREBP	sterol-regulatory element binding protein
SRSA	slow-reacting substance of anaphylaxis
SS	signs & symptoms
SSBG	sex steroid binding globulin (AKA SHBG)
SSRI	selective serotonin reuptake inhibitor
StAR	**steroidogenic acute regulatory protein; rate-limiting enzyme of steroidogenesis**
STAT	signal transducers activators of transcription
subcut	subcutaneous
supf	superficial
SV	seminal vesicles

SymNS   sympathetic nervous system

T

T	tissue
T3	triiodothyronine
T4	thyroxine
TAG	triacylglyceride, triacylglycerol
TAK1	**transforming growth factor-β-activated kinase 1**
TAT	**tyrosine aminotransferase**
TGA	therapeutic goods administration
TBG	thyroid binding globulin (binds TH in the B)
TCR	T-cell antigen receptor
TED	thyroid eye disease AKA Grave's ophthalmopathy
TEL	telomere
TFII	**transcription factors that regulate the activity of RNA polymerase II**
TFM	testicular feminization syndrome
TFPI	tissue factor pathway inhibitor
TGA/TG	triglyceride
TGF	transforming growth factor
TH	non specific thyroid H made up of T_3 & T_4
THF	tetrahydrofolate
THP	**tryptophan hydroxylase**
TNF	tumor necrosis factor, α & β
TNF-α	tumor necrosis factor-α
TNF-β	tumor necrosis factor-β
tPA	tissue plasmogen activator
TPP	thiamine pyrophosphate
TPO	thyroid peroxidase
TR	thyroid hormone receptor
TRF	thyrotropin-releasing factor AKA thyroid hormone releasing hormone (TRH)
tRNA	transfer RNA / transport RNA
TSAb	thyroid stimulating autoantibodies; bind to TSH receptor mimicking TSH action, leads to hyperthyroidism of Graves disease
TSH	thyroid-stimulating hormone
TSI	thyroid stimulating immunoglobulins
Tx	treatment
TX	thromboxane
TZD	thiazolidinedione

U

| UCD | urea cycle disorder |
| UCP1 | uncoupling protein 1, AKA thermogenin |

V

V	veins
v	very
VCAM	vascular cell adhesion molecule
VDR	vitamin D receptor
VEGF	vascular endothelial growth factor
VHL	von-Hippel-Lindau syndrome
VIP	vasoactive intestinal peptide
Vita	vitamin
VLCFA	very long-chain fatty acid
VLCS	**very long-chain acyl-CoA synthetase**; AKA **FA transport protein**
VLDL	very low density lipoprotein
VMN	ventromedial nucleus; hypothalamic region involved in satiety (sensation of being full)
VSGP	vertical supranuclear gaze palsy
vWF	von Willebrand factor

W

WAT	white adipose tissue
w/n	within
w/o	without
wrt	with respect to

X

| XP | xeroderma pigmentosum |

V

ZF	zona fasciculata
ZG	zona glomerulosa
ZR	zona reticularis
&	and
ω	omega

Pronunciation Key & Colour Guide

Most terms are listed in black

Pathological terms are in green

Prefixes and Suffixes are in blue

Endocrine / Vitamin terms in maroon

The pronunciation guide to words in this section are in bold red lettering

Stressed syllables are in **CAPITAL LETTERS**

Vowel sounds are pronounced as indicated below

A	May	ay
	map	a
	mark	ah
E	Me	ee
	met	e
	term	ur
I	eye / sight	ï
	tin	i
O	go	oh
	mother	uh
	mop	o
	more	or
	boy	oi
	lose	oo
	nook	oe
	loose	ou
U	blue	ou
	cute	ew
	cut	uh
Y	family	ee
	myth	i
	eye	ï

Common Terms used in Endocrinology

A

a- without, lack of, no

ab- away from, negative

Abdomen *Lt. abdomen = the belly*, the part of the trunk b/n thorax & the perineum,

Aberrant *Lt. ab = from*, & *errare = to wander*, hence, deviating from normal.

Absorption (ab-SORB-shun) the passage of material, such as an embryo, from a lumen of an organ into another body space, T or cell

ac- toward, near to, addition to

Accessory *Lt. accessum = added*, hence, supplementary.

Acetyl CoA AKA Acetylcoenzyme A is the precursor for cholesterol synthesis. It is made up of an acetyl grp **(1)** + co-Enzyme A **(2)** which has 2 components Pantothenic acid - Vita B5 **(3)** & phosphorylated ADP **(4)**. All carbon molecules in the human are derived from the 2 carbons in the acetyl grp **(1)** *(see also Coenzymes)*

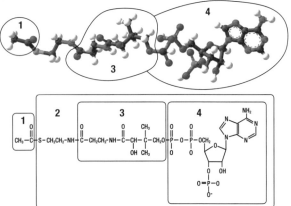

Achalasia (AY-kal-ay-si-ya) failure of relaxation of smooth muscle

Acini (AS-i-nee) clusters of cells which face a lumen and are often parts of an exocrine gland that secrete digestive enzymes. *sing. acinus (AS-in-us) adj. acinar*

Acne (AK-nee) *Gk: acme = point or achne = to chaff* an inflammatory condition of the pilosebacious unit – hair unit in the skin - exacerbated by progesterone in the female & reduced by oestrogen

acu- sudden, sharp , severe

© A. L. Neill

Acute (AK-yewt) – *Gk: acu- acus = needle sharp*, sudden onset + short course pathological process – used to describe any condition which starts suddenly & is of short duration; may be associated with a sharp needle-like pain of relatively short duration ≠ chronic, although 2 separate processes, they may co-exist.

ad- near, toward

Addison's disease AKA Chronic Adrenal Insufficiency AKA Hypoadrenalism characterised by abdominal pains, hypotension, & weakness. When under stress the disease may become an Addisonian crisis resulting in coma, due to severe drop in BP, & death.

aden- gland

Adenoid: *Gk. aden = a gland, eidos = shape or form.*

Adenohypophysis AKA the Anterior Lobe of the Pituitary Gland. It is composed of glandular epithelium. The adenohypophysis secretes numerous Hs, several of which affect the activity of other endocrine glands, including the reproductive organs/glands.

Adequate Intake (AI) when there is no established RDA the alternative is a measure of the adequate intake of a Vita mineral or other essential substance

Adipogenesis the synthesizing of fats & AT

Adipokine AKA Adipocytokine proteins secreted by AT which modulate a range of pathological, physiological & metabolic activities both globally & locally e.g. appetite control, E balance, lipid metabolism, glucose homeostasis, IF, angiogenesis, regulation of B coagulation & BP, inflammatory mediator stimulation

Adipose (AD-i-pohs) *Lt. adeps = fat, hence fatty* used to describe a CT whose cells (adipocytes) are highly specialized for lipid storage *see Fat tissue, White Adipose Tissue (WAT).*

Adolescence the transition of childlike mental development to adult reasoning coincident with puberty

adeno- pertaining to glands see also glands

Adrenal (AD-reen-al): *Lt. ad = towards, at, ren = kidney*, situated near the kidney (AKA suprarenal) *adj. adrenergic Gk. ergon = work*, stimuli which cause the adrenal (suprarenal) gland to produce adrenaline; also indicates Ns or pathways which use adrenalin as a transmitter.

Adrenarche (ad-ren-ARK-ee) is an early sexual maturation stage, b/n 10 - 11yo. The adrenal cortex secretes ↑ androgens e.g. DHEA, but w/o ↑ cortisol, from the new cortical zone ZR. Although related to puberty it is distinct from the hypothalamic – pituitary – gonadal axis.

aero- air, pertaining to gas

af- near, toward, addition to

agglut- (a-GLOOT) to glue

Aging is the progressive ↓ of physiological functions that ↑ the probability of death. Functional decline occurs w/n the cells, particularly the "permanent cells" which do not undergo mitosis after formation e.g.: cerebral neural T; skeletal & cardiac muscle; and kidney cells. Cells which constantly multiply throughout life show very few signs of aging e.g.: blood & intestinal epithelium. In the skin it is the fibrous dermis which contributes the most to the aging process, while the epithelium remains relatively unaffected.

Percentage of normal T &/or function left in the average elderly person (>75yo)	%
Brain weight	56
Cerebral BS	80
CO at rest	70
Number of functioning glomeruli / kidney function	56
GFR	69
Acid/Base recovery after displacement	17
Number of functioning taste buds	36
Vital capacity	56
Strength of hand grip	55
Maximum O_2 uptake during exercise	40
Number of axons in spinal nerve	63
Velocity of nerve impulse	90
Body weight	88

Alicyclic (AL-ee-sï-klik) curved; C to C bonds in an aromatic ring are shared & curved going around the ring, so that each C to C bond is actually 1.5 bonds with the central bonds not aligned to a particular C. This property allows the ring to absorb UV light, & is seen in the aromatic AAs. (≠ **aliphatic**).

alipo- pertaining to fat

Aliphatic (AL-ee-fat-ik) straight; C to C linear bonds are aliphatic, generally used to describe a long straight hydrocarbon chain. They may be single, saturated bonds or they may be double, unsaturated bonds capable of reacting with other molecules or radicals & expanding (≠ **alicyclic**).

Allantois: Gk. allantos = sausage, eidos = like, form.

amin(o)- an organic substance containing nitrogen

Ammonia is a by-product of deamination, usually from AAs when used as fuel in the body. Ammonia is toxic & must be converted to an inert nitrogen-containing-compound - urea - the main organic waste product of the body. This occurs in the liver and then urea is excreted by the kidneys

Ammonia

Urea

© A. L. Neill

Anabolism reactions which build up molecules & use E (≠ **catabolism**)

Androgen AKA Androgenic H AKA Testoid the broad term for any natural or synthetic compound, that stimulates or controls the development & maintenance of male sexual characteristics e.g. testosterone, dihydrotestosterone (DHT) which is responsible for the development of the scrotum & testis and later prostate growth & male pattern baldness.

Andropause male equivalent of menopause with ↓ testosterone

Anorexigenic appetite suppressing (≠ **orexogenic**)

Anions negatively charged atoms or radicals e.g. Cl-, OH-

ante- (AN-tee) before

anti- against, combating

Antibody / Antigen, proteins involved in the immune system – antibodies *Abs* are produced by the body in reaction to antigens *Ags* proteins or materials found on the surface of FBs introduced to the body forming the Ab/Ag complex.

AutoAbs are those Abs which develop against the *Ags* of the host - i.e. autoimmune e.g. after a vasectomy the body may develop *AutoAbs* against sperm, & *AutoAbs* are commonly implicated in thyroid disease, Grave's disease and Hashimoto's disease.

Apocrine secretions which take off the cytoplasm of the apex of the cell as well

Apolipoprotein AKA Apoprotein a protein which binds lipids together to form lipoproteins & / or chylomicrons lipid cells which wrap around lipid materials enabling them to be transported through the BS protecting them from the watery contents.

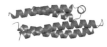

Apoptysis (AP-pop-te-sis) *Gk aptos = to drop out* describes pockets of dead or dying cells - found in all organs wedged b/n healthy cells so it is thought to be a physiological phenomenon of normal aging or cellular weeding out *AKA programmed cell death* e.g. in the liver & ovary.

Arachidonic acid (a-RAK-id-on-ik) AKA Icosanoic acid AKA Eicosanoic cold (Ī-KOS-an-oh-ic) is a polyunsaturated ω-6 20-Carbon FA, It has 3 unsaturated bonds. Its saturated equivalent is arachidic acid found in peanuts but this FA is not found in plants.

It is present in the phospholipids of the cms throughout the body & particularly abundant in brain, muscles & liver. SKM retains 20% of the body's total store. Here it is responsible for the growth, maintenance & repair of that T, e.g. after exercise. It is the main precursor of the synthesis of the eicosanoids whose subfamilies include the PGs, powerful pro-If Hs. When liberated via the destruction of the cm it stimulates If & IMR, directly & via its metabolites.

Argentaffin cells cells which take up silver stains when prepared for histology e.g. enteroendocrine cells, which have H granules capable of being stained with silver *see also Enteroendocrine cells*

Asthenia unusual fatigability & weakness as seen in Addison's disease AKA Chronic adrenal insufficiency

asthen- weak, weakness

Atopy (AY-top-ee) *Gk atopis = out of place* group of diseases characterized by the tendency to have a severe hypersensitive reaction to common materials as in the RT, GIT & skin *adj. atopy* = allergic as in atopic dermatitis = skin If

auto- (OR-toh) self, spontaneous

Autocrine secretions of the cell influence other like cells & its own function

Autolysis (OR-tol-e-sis) *Gk auto = self, lysis = dissolving* - hence the process of self destruction of a cell or tissue

aux- (ORKS) help, growth, increase

B

Bartholin's glands AKA Greater Vestibular Glands

bary- low, heavy, deep difficult

Basement membrane AKA Basal lamina (BM) a thin layer of extracellular material & CT stroma that underlies every epithelium.

basi- foundation, base

baso- base c.f. acid / base & in the bottom – the basal layer

bio- (bĭ-oh) life

Biogenesis the development or formation of ...e.g. biogenesis of an organelle may result from the fusion of several components ± their further modification

Borborygmi (BOR-bor-rig-me) stomach grumbling

Break-through -bleeding bleeding in the middle of the menstral cycle which indicates irregular H levels - if the person is on OCs it indicates a need for adjustment of these Hs - generally a reduction in the progesterone levels &/or ⬆ oestrogen levels

Brown fat AKA Brown adipose tissue small part of AT as a whole concentrated around the central organs more important in the neonate

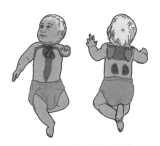

C

Capsule (KAPS-yew-l) *Lt. capsa = box*, hence an enclosing membrane

Carcinogen (KAR-sin-oh-jen) material which leads to cancer formation

Carcinoma (KAR-sin-oh-mah) a malignant growth originating from epithelial cells

Carcinoma – *in situ* pre-invasive cancer still lying in the confines of normal tissue not having broken through the BM but with neoplastic changes, e.g. in the cervix

Castration (CAS-tray-shon) removal of the genitalia generally in ref. to the male - note if the prostate gland remains it is still possible to have an orgasm. In the female castration is the removal of the ovaries, which does not interfere with the ability to orgasm. **Casterati** - young boys castrated to preserve their voice & maintain their physique.

Catabolism reactions which break down substances & produce E (≠ **anabolism**)

Catecholamine (KAT-e-kohl-ay-meen) an organic compound with a ***"catechol"* (1)** which is a BENZENE RING + 2 hydroxyl side groups & an amine side-chain; a monoamine, derived from Tyrosine **(2)** or via hydroxylation of Phenylalanine. Catecholamines are water-soluble & 50%-bound to plasma proteins in the BS. The 3 Hs which are catecholamines are: adrenaline **(3)**, dopamine **(5)** & noradrenaline **(4)**.

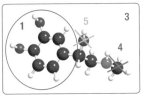
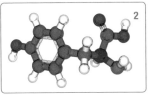

Catamenia (KAT-uh-meen-ee-yuh) AKA Menses AKA Menstruation
Gk Katamenios = monthly

Caveolin membrane-bound proteins involved in receptor-dependant endocytosis *pl caveolae*

Cell (SELL) the basic living unit of multi-cellular organisms.

Cell body AKA SOMA the portion of a neuron containing the nucleus & much of the cytoplasm.

Cell membrane (cm) AKA plasma membrane the bilipid membrane layer & its associated proteins surrounding the cell & separating it from the outside, w/n the cell several areas are compartmentalized via similar membranes e.g. ER, GA, the nucleus, liposomes & vacuoles- *(see also nuclear membrane)*

cer- (ser) wax

ceramide *Lt. cera = wax* are a family of waxy lipid molecules **(B)**, composed of sphingosines **(A)** & FAs. The FA residue **(1)** binds to the sphingosine to give the aliphatic chain **(2)** some hydrophilic properties. They are found in high concentrations w/n the cm bilipid layer. Ceramides participate in a variety of cellular e.g. regulating differentiation, proliferation & cell death.

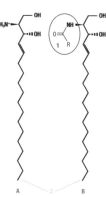

chaperones molecules which assist in a protein to "fold" correctly into its bioactive shape from its native shape, while preventing aggregation & intermolecular bonding *(see also protein folding)*

chemo- relating to chemistry, chemically induced (keem-oh)

Chemosis is oedema of the conjunctiva, due to the exudation from inflamed permeable capillaries. It may be a nonspecific sign of eye irritation, or due to AI disease generally assoc. with hyperthyroidism. The conjunctiva becomes swollen & may appear gelatinous, with the eyeball unable to be fully covered by the eyelid. This can result in drying of the cornea, scarring, & visual disturbances.

Chemotaxis (KEEM-oh-tax-is) cellular phenomenon of moving towards or away from specific areas due to the chemical present

Chloasma (KLOH-az-muh) AKA Melasma hyperpigmentation of the sensitive areas of the skin exposed to sunlight due to H imbalance often ↑ LH (as in pregnancy).

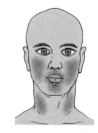

Chromatin (KROH-mah-tin) the mass of genetic material in the nucleus of a cell, consisting mostly of DNA. It is only visible during interphase.

Chromosome (KRO-moh-sohm) one of the structures (46 in human cells) w/n the cell nucleus that contains genetic material. Chromosomes become visible during cell division.

chron- time (kron-)

Chronic (KRON-ik) long standing, generally used in disease states (≠ **acute**)

Chronic Adrenal Insufficiency AKA Addison's disease

chyle- digested fats (KĬ-l) *Gk. = juice.*

Chiral asymmetrical - the property of a C atom which has 4 different bonds, to "rotate" the plane of polarized light in a particular direction - i.e. this is the "handedness" of the molecule, Rotation of the light to the LEFT is **levorotatory.**
All natural AAs are levorotatory (except Glycine, which is symmetrical). Some ABs rotate light to the RIGHT, **dextrorotatory**.

Cholesterol (KOHL-est-er-ol) *Gk. chole = bile steros = solid ol = alcohol* $C_{27}H_{46}O$ - an essential organic modified steroid used in cm, bile salts & as a precursor for steroid Hs & Vita D synthesis.

cine- (sin-ee) movement

Climateric AKA Menopause

coen- general , common

Coenzymes AKA Co-substrates e.g. vitamins, small, organic non-protein molecules, which carry chemical groups b/n enzymes, although they are not part of the enzyme's structure. One of the most common is Co-enzyme A, used to form cholesterol and made up of **1**- cysteine (an AA) + **2**- pantothenate + **3**- phosphate groups + **4**- ribose (a sugar) + 5- adenine (a nucleotide) *see also cofactor & cholesterol formation*

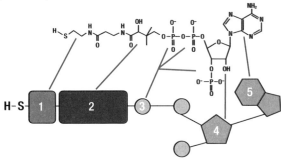

col- with, together

coelom- (SEE-lohm) body cavity

Cofactors AKA Helper molecules (1) non-protein chemical compounds, bound to the protein **(2)** & necessary for its biological activity **(3)** e.g. its ability to catabolise **(5)** a substrate **(4)**. There are two types of cofactors:

Coenzymes, cofactors loosely bound to the enzyme &

Prosthetic groups, cofactors bound tightly to the enzyme. An enzyme w/o a cofactor is an apoenzyme **(2a)** & a "complete" enzyme is an holoenzyme **(2h)**.

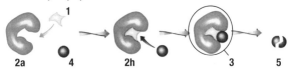

Connective tissue (kon-EK-tiv Tishh-ew) (CT) one of the 4 basic types of tissue in the body. It is characterized by an abundance of EC material with relatively few cells, and functions in the support & binding of body structures.

contra- opposite against

Corpus: *Lt. = body, pl.- corpora.* pertaining to the body or the main part of the organ

Corpus luteum (KOR-puhs-LOO-tee-uhm) (CL) a structure w/n the ovary that forms from a ruptured Graäfian follicle & functions as an endocrine gland by secreting female Hs.

Corpuscle (KOR-puhs-ehl) *Lt. = a little body* hence used to describe a small body contained w/n a sac, as in red corpuscle (RBC) small package of haemoglobin

Cortex (KOR-tehks) *Lt. = bark, adj. cortical* the outer portion of an organ. (≠ **medulla**)

cost- (kost) rib *Lt. = rib. adj.- costal*

Crenation (kre-NAY-shun) the shrinkage of a cell caused by contact with an hypotonic solution.

Crescent (KRES-ent) crown of epithelial cells – as seen in glomerulonephritis on Bowman's capsule or around the discharged ovum

-crine (krïn) to secrete

Cushing's syndrome AKA Hypercortisolism is caused by an excess of cortisol or cortisol-like substances, SS include: hypertension, central obesity with thin arms & legs, stretch marks & fragile skin from weakened collagen, weak SKM & poor healing.

cutis - (KEW-tis) skin

Cutaneous (kew-TAY-nee-us) *adj Lt. cutis = skin* the skin.

Cytochrome are proteins containing haeme groups where iron is fixed in the centre responsible for the generation of ATP. They are found either as monomeric proteins e.g. cytochrome C or as subunits of bigger enzymatic complexes e.g. Haemoglobin that catalyze redox reactions. They direct the oxidation/reduction of oxygen in these reactions, & there are at least 20,000 different forms.

Cytochrome P450 group AKA CYPs
(1) are involved in providing E for anabolic reactions w/n the cell & are fixed to the SER &/or mitochondrial inner membrane. They do this using the porphyrin ring **(2)** containing a ferrous ion (Fe^{2+}) **(3)** The P450 is derived from its maximum peak wavelength absorption (450 nm)

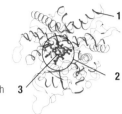

cyt-/-cyte (sït-) cell mature cell type

Cytokine *Gk. cyto = cell, kine = movement.* a protein signalling molecule i.e. a broad category of small cell-signalling proteins released by a large variety of cells to affect the behaviour of other cells. They mainly affect the immune system, & may act on other cytokines. They differ from Hs in that they need much higher concentrations to be effective & are not as cell specific i.e. many cell types may produce the same cytokine. But there is an overlap in terminology with cytokines referred to as Hs e.g. Erythropoietin. Generally Hs can only be produced by one or 2 cell types.

Cytoplasm (SĪ-to-plazm) the material of a cell located w/n the cm & outside the nm, containing the cellular organelles.

Cytosol (SĪ-toh-sol) the thickened fluid of the cytoplasm. It lies outside the cellular organelle membranes.

Cytoskeleton (SĪ-toh-SKEL-eh-ton) the complex supportive network of microtubules & microfilaments in the cytoplasm.

D

Deamination the removal of the amine grp (NH_2) from AAs to form ammonia (NH_3) & ketone acids *see also Ammonia*.

Deciduation shedding of endometrial T during menstruation.

Degeneration - retrogressive cell & T changes short of necrosis

Dendrite: or dendron, *Gk. = a tree*, hence like the branches of a tree.

dendro- branching, treelike

Deoxyribonucleic acid (dee-ox-see-rï-boh-nyoo-KLAY-ik A-sid) (DNA) nucleic acids in the shape of a double helix containing the genetic information necessary for protein synthesis. The outer proteins **(2)** protect the inner base codes **(1)** - when unravelled the bases expose a code for specific proteins - Hs and other substances. Proteins binding onto the surface of the helix **(3)** also influence which proteins can and cannot be synthesized. These outer proteins have been implicated in the formation of uncontrolled growth - neoplasms.

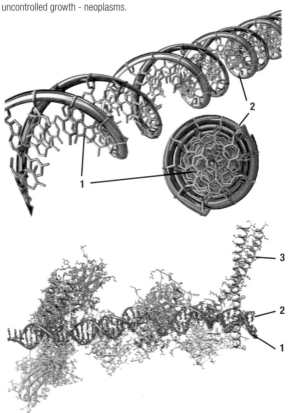

Dermis (DER-mis) *Gk. = skin, adj.- dermal* the layer of the skin lying deep to the epidermis & composed of dense irregular CT. The collagen fibres are maintained by female Hs particularly oestrogen. After the menopause collagen fibres breakdown & the skin appears frailer & translucent as the dermis is reduced.

Differentiation (DIF-er-ent-she-ay-shon) the process of changing from one kind of T or cell to another, generally to a more complex form.

diplo- double, twin

dis- apart from, two, twice, double , reversal, separation, difficult, wrong

Dipsogen *Gk. dypsa = thirst & gen = to create* an agent that causes thirst.

duo- (DEW-oh) two

E

Effluvian (EH-floo-vee-an) shedding of hair, may occur in times of stress &/or due to H changes e.g.: andropause, menopause & pregnancy. Generally hair regrows after months but this is not always the case

Eicosanoids AKA Icosanoids. (Ī-kos-an-oyd) are a varied group of pro-IF signalling molecules found throughout the body derived from the oxidation of polyunsaturated FAs e.g. arachidonic acid. They are involved in controlling cellular activity e.g. growth assoc with the IF &/or immune processes, & have several classes e.g. the PGs & their derivatives: prostacyclins, lipoxins, & thromboxanes; & the LTs. Their half life is extremely short and their effect, local, being either autocrine or paracrine. NSAIDs & antioxidants attack either the formation or levels of eicosanoids *see also Arachidonic acid*

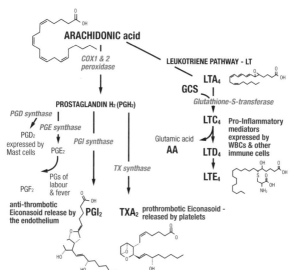

Metabolic actions of selected eicosanoids			
PGD_2	Promotion of sleep	TXA_2	Stimulation of platelet aggregation; vasoconstriction
PGE_2	Smooth muscle contraction; inducing pain, heat, fever; bronchoconstriction	15d-PGJ_2	Adipocyte differentiation
$PGF_{2\alpha}$	Uterine contractions	LTB_4	Leukocyte chemotaxis
PGI_2	Inhibition of platelet aggregation; vasodilation, embryo implanatation	Cysteinyl-LTs	Anaphylaxis; bronchial smooth muscle contraction.
† Shown eicosanoids are AA-derived; in general, EPA-derived have weaker activity			

en- within, inside, in, on

endo- within, inside, into, on

Endocrine: (EN-do-krin) *Gk. endo = within : krinein = to separate*, organs/cells that secrete products directly into the BS, generally glands secreting Hs

Endosomes membrane-bound body in the cell generally from ingested material & requiring further digestion – a progression in the path to lysosome differentiation *see also Lysosome, Vesicle*

Endoplasmic reticulum (en-doh-PLAZ-mik reh-TIK-yew-lum) (ER) a cytoplasmic organelle that consists of a series of tubules with a hollow center. It functions in the transport of cellular products (smooth ER - SER), & as a site for protein synthesis (if ribosomes are attached, called rough ER - RER).

Endorphins AKA Endogenous morphine are endogenous opioid inhibitory neuropeptides. They are produced by the CNS & Pituitary gland. Endorphins are responsible for a pharmaceutical activity &/or emotional response rather than specific chemical formulations.

Endothelium (en-doh-THEE-lee-um) *Gk. endo = within, & thele = the nipple* a layer of simple squamous epithelium lining the inside of BVs & the heart chambers.

Enteroendocrine cells sometimes called Argentaffin cells are specialized group of endocrine cells of the GIT & pancreas, which produce GIT Hs or peptides, mainly seratonin. Their secretions often stimulate the peristalsis of the gut, or the secretions of digestive enzymes. The basal cells lie on the BM **(1)**, protected by the epithelial lining cells **(2)** & secrete their Hs **(4)** based upon the gut's contents & volume into the surrounding BS **(3)**.

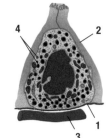

-ergy (er-jee) action

erythr- (er-RITH) red

Erythropoiesis the synthesis of erythrocytes AKA RBCs

eso- (EE-soh) within

Ester bond the combination of an alcohol's hydroxyl group with an organic acid's carboxyl group. Many substances form multiple bonds e.g. TGs **(1)** are made up of glycerol **(2)** (which has 3 hydroxy (-OH) grps) **(5)** combining with saturated **(3i)** or unsaturated **(3ii, 3iii,4)** FAs**(3)** (each one with a carboxyl grp -COOH) **(7)** forming a TG.+ 3 molecules of water **(8)**, one for each bond formed *see also TG*

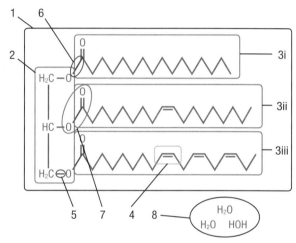

Estrue AS Oestrue refers to a female animal on heat *i.e. the animal is in estrue*

eu- good normal well easily

eury- broad wide

Euthyroid (yoo-THĬ-royd) normal TH levels

exo- outside outer layer out of

Exocrine (EK-soh-krin) gland, one of two main categories of glands, here the cellular products are released into ducts then transported to a body surface or into a body cavity.

extra- outside of; out, over, beyond, in addition to,

Extracellular environment (EKS-trah-CEL-yew-lar en-VĬ-ROH-ment) the body space outside the cm of cells.

Extracellular fluid (ECF) the fluid outside the cm of cells, including interstitial fluid & B plasma.

F

Factor AKA Hormone

Fat in human biology this is a TG, a subgroup of lipids. The universal structure is 3 long chain FAs bound together by glycerol, the components of which vary with diet, *see also Triglycerides (TGs)*.

Fat tissue AKA white adipose T (WAT) loose highly vascularized, highly innervated CT consisting of large adipocytes containing a single lipid vacuole >90% of the total volume of the cell, *more detail in the text*.

Fatty acid (FA) is a carboxylic acid with a long aliphatic chain. If the bonds b/n the carbon & the hydrogen are all single then the FA is *saturated* **(1)**. If there are any double bonds on the carbon atoms then the FA is *unsaturated* **(2)** & has the potential to covalently bind to further atoms.

With the *unsaturated* FAs they may be a "straight" line & hence they are *trans FAs* or "curved" then *cis* FAs **(3)**. Trans FAs rarely occur in natural oils or fats. **Free Fatty Acids** (FFAs) are those FAs which are not bound to glycerol or other carrier substance. FAs are named according to the position of the first 2X bond counting from the methyl end.

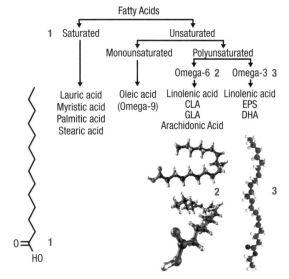

Fatty Acids

```
                          Fatty Acids
                               |
       ┌───────────────────────┴───────────────────────┐
1   Saturated                              Unsaturated
                          ┌──────────────────┴──────────────────┐
                   Monounsaturated                    Polyunsaturated
                                                  ┌──────────┴──────────┐
                                              Omega-6 2          Omega-3 3

   Lauric acid        Oleic acid      Linolenic acid       Linolenic acid
   Myristic acid      (Omega-9)           CLA                   EPS
   Palmitic acid                          GLA                   DHA
   Stearic acid                     Arachidonic Acid
```

Fight or Flight response AKA Fight, flight, Freeze or Fawn response AKA Hyperarousal AKA Acute Stress response is a physiological reaction that occurs in response to a perceived threat. It is the reaction of a general discharge of the SymNS, which also involves the adrenal medulla & secretion of the catecholamines, which act as post ganglionic sympathetic

© A. L. Neill

Ns. Oestrogen & Testosterone and Dopamine & Serotonin are also involved in the acute stress response. Many of the reactions of the Fight or Flight are mediated by adrenaline & noradrenaline either via the adrenal medulla ± SymNS, and these are:

↑↑ HR BP BF to the muscles and away from the GIT, B[sugar], B[FFAs], tremor, lipolysis, reflexes, pupil size

↓↓ peripheral vision, tear production

Other reactions are mediated by the adrenal cortex Hs - particularly in long term stress reactions, as the body changes and adapts to stress.

Formication sensation of crawling under the skin often associated with menopause, associated with ↓ Dopamine.

Foam cell a resident T macrophage **(1)** which is filled with lipid, which it has taken from circulating VLDLs, closely associated with the BVs in this case a capillary **(2)**. The lipid droplets are placed in residual bodies which look like foam **(3)**.

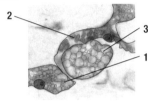

Free radicals unbound charged ions or molecules - highly reactive *see also Radicals*

G

Gamete (ga-MEET) a sex cell. It may be male (spermatozoa) or female (oocyte).

γ gamma: *the 3rd letter of the Gk. alphabet*, used in sequence - α -alpha, β - beta, γ -gamma, δ - delta, etc. until ω - omega

Ganglion (GANG-lee-on) *Gk. = swelling adj.- ganglionic* a cluster of neuron cell bodies located outside the CNS.

Gemellus: *Lt. diminutive of geminus = twin.*

Gene (JEEN) functional unit of hereditary occupying a specific place on a chromosome, which directs the formation of a specific protein

-genesis the creation of; the formation of, the building up of , the synthesis of..

Gestational Diabetes AKA Diabetes of pregnancy

Gland *Lt. glans = an acorn, adj.- glandular* a specialization of epithelial T to secrete substances. It may consist of a single cell or a multicellular arrangement

Glucocorticoids (GLOO-koh-kor-tik-oyds) substances which raise the levels of B[sugar]. The most abundant glucocorticoid is ***cortisol (AKA hydrocortisone)***. They also have potent anti-If effects.

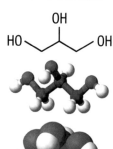

Glycan (GLĬ-kan) a sugar

Glycosylation (GLĬ-kos-ee-LAY-shon) attachment of 1 or more sugars to a molecule

Glycerol (GLIS-er-ol) AKA Glycerine AS Glycerin is a sugar alcohol, with 3 hydroxyl groups, making it soluble in water, viscous and hygroscopic in that it draws water to it. It readily forms ester bonds with organic acids and it forms the backbone of all lipids known as triglycerides (TG).

Glycolation (GLĬ-koh-lay-shon) the spontaneous random formation of proteins or lipids with circulating sugars. This occurs with increased sugar levels as in DM and can be used as a measure of B[sugar]. It also ↑ with age. *(see also Glycosylation)*

Glycoproteins proteins with covalently attached CHOs

Glycosylation (GLĬ-koz-ee-lay-shon) the precise enzymatic formation of covalent bonds b/n proteins &/or other biological substances & sugars to make them biologically more hydrophilic. For example this ceramide **(1)** has enhanced hydrophilia with the sugar attached **(2)** making it a cerebroside **(3)**.

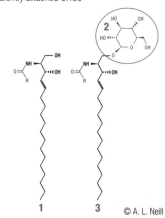

© A. L. Neill

Goitre AKA Goiter (GOY-the) an enlargement of the thyroid gland *(2)*, ranging from a small lump to a huge mass, which may cause swallowing & breathing problems because it affects the trachea **(3)** or presses on the cricoid cartilage **(1)**.

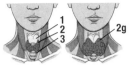

Most goitres **(2g)** are caused by iodine deficiency (~90%) & thyroid conditions, such as hyperthyroidism, hypothyroidism, nodules & cancer.

gon- sexual

Gonad (GOH-nad) *Gk. = reproduction adj. - gonadal* an organ that produces gametes & sex Hs. ♂. = the testes; ♀. = the ovaries.

Gonadarche the earliest gonadal changes of puberty, in response to pituitary gonadotropins. The ovaries & testes begin to ↑ in size & & ↑ the production of sex Hs; oestrogen & testosterone. *see also Menarche & Thelarche*

Gonadotophin AS Gonadotropin (US) Hs to promote the growth of gonads or sex organs & maintain 2° sexual characteristics

goni- corner

gnos – *Gk: gnos = to know* **(nos)** *agnos = not to know* **(AG-nos)**

Graves' disease an autoimmune disorder associated with the presence of thyroid-stimulating immunoglobulins (TSI) AKA TSH receptor antibodies **(1a)**. These Abs mimic TSH **(1)** bind to the TSH receptor **(2)** more firmly than the H & stimulate the thyroid cells **(3)** continuously, releasing high levels of THs **(4)** so the patient develops a form of thyrotoxicosis AKA hyperthyroidism. It occurs in 1:500 pregnancies. SS include: anxiety, diarrhoea, fatigue, goitre, heat intolerance, irritability, nervousness, pretibial myoedema, tachycardia, tremors, weakness & weight loss see also ***Graves' Ophthalmopathy AKA Thyroid Eye Disease in the main text***

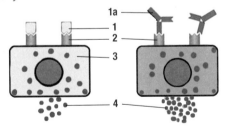

Gynaecomastica development of male breast T, present in prepubescent boys but tends to regress with puberty. Re-emerges with age & ↑ wgt & particular medications including alcohol, which ↑ the levels of circulating oestrogens.

H

Haeme AKA heme (HEEM) is a cofactor consisting of an Fe^{2+} **(1)** (ferrous) ion contained in the centre of a large heterocyclic organic ring - a porphyrin **(2)**. This is then associated with a large protein to couple with its redox reactions either as a single monomeric or multiple units making them haemoproteins. The commonest is haemoglobin but they are also part of the cytochrome protein system e.g. in the P450 cytochromes.

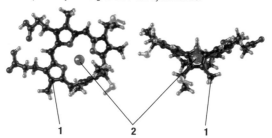

1   2   1

Haemoproteins proteins containing the ferrous ion.

Hashimoto thyroiditis AKA Hashimoto's disease AKA goitrous chronic thyroiditis. an autoimmune disease with thyroid peroxidase Ab (anti-TPO), an autoAb against *thyroid peroxidase enzyme*. Many patients also have anti-thyroglobulin Abs. The resulting symptoms are those of hypothyroidism. The disease often follows Grave's disease, & is similar to **postpartum thyroiditis (PPT)**

hidr- sweat

Hidrosis (HĬ-droh-sis) disease of the sweat glands

holo- entire

Holocrine secretions which involve the death of the cell with substance liberation

homo- same

homeo (HOHM-ee-oh) same common like

Homeostasis (HOH-me-oh-stay-sis) condition of cells in organs or T where loss of the units (cells usually) is equal to the formation of new units

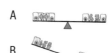

horm- to urge to stimulate

Hormone (H) (HOR-mohn) a substance secreted by endocrine T that changes the physiological activity of the target cell.

Hot Flushes *see Vasomotor instability*

hydr- (hïdr) water

Hypercortisolism AKA Cushing's syndrome

Hypocortisolism AKA Addison's disease

Hypophysis AKA Pituitary (Hï-poh-fif-sis) *Gk. hypo = down, physis = growth*, hence, a down growth (from the brain). However, this is not the whole truth. Part is an upward growth from the pharynx, *adj.- hypophysial*.

Hypomenorrhea AKA Scanty periods

Hypothalamus (hï-poh-THAL-u-mus) *Gk. hypo = under, and thalamus* the small, inferior portion of the diencephalon in the brain. It functions mainly in the control of involuntary activities, including endocrine gland regulation, sleep, thirst & hunger.

hyster- (hister-) uterine

Hystero *Gk = hyster to do with the uterus* thought to be the seat of all female emotion hence hysterical

I

iatr- (ee-at-rah) to treat

Icosanoic acid AKA Arachidonic acid

ictero- (IK-ter-oh) jaundiced

im- in, into, on, onto, not, non

In vitro (ihn VEE-tro) outside the body, such as in a culture bottle.

In vivo (ihn VEE-vo) inside the living body.

Infundibulum (in-fun-DIB-yoo-lum) *Lt. = funnel* the narrow connection b/n the hypothalamus of the brain & the pituitary gland, also, the funnel-shaped distal end of the uterine tube which opens near an ovary.

insul- island

inter - between

Intercellular (in-ter-SEL-yoo-lar) the area b/n cells.

Interstitial cells (in-ter-STIH-shul) cells b/n lobes or structures in an organ e.g. in the testes they are located b/n seminiferous tubules that secrete testosterone, *AKA Leydig cells*.

Interstitial fluid (ihn-tehr-STIH-shool FLOO-id) the portion of ec fluid which fills the T spaces b/n cells. (see also = tissue fluid & intercellular fluid).

Ions - charged atoms ***see also Free Radicals***
   -ve charge - anions - generally non-metal
   +ve charge - cations generally metal

Isoelectric point (pI) the pH at which the average net charge of a molecule e.g. an AA is zero *see also Zwitterion*.

K

ketone bodies (KBs) are the product of protein deamination, when protein is broken down for food, eg acetone **(1)**, acetoacid **(2)** & β-hydroxybutyric acid **(3)**.

-kine- move

-kines stimulation of activation for division or growth of cells

L

Lamina propria (LP) proper layer, background T surrounding major specialized cell masses in an organ - often loose areolar T: a combination of CT, immune cells, BVs, lymphocytes & Ns

Leydig's cells AKA interstitial cells of the testis.

leio- (LĪ-oh) smooth

Libido (lib-EE-doh) AKA sex drive the urge & interest in having sex

Ligand is a molecule that binds a metal atom **(1)** to the centre of a protein & forms a coordination complex, fixing it in a specific position via e- bonds e.g. in haem - Histadine **(2)**, acts as a ligand binding the Fe **(1)** in the centre of the protein, surrounded by AA helices **(3)** & AA chains

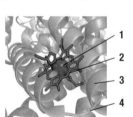

Lipoproteins AKA Chylomicrons

Luteum (LOO-tee-um) adj. Lt. = yellow.

ly- dissolved

Lymph (LIMpf) excess fluid & proteins left behind from the capillaries as they move from the arterial to the venous side

M

Macrophage (mØ) (MAK-roh-fahrj) a large phagocytic cell originating from a monocyte.

macula: *Lt. = spot* (cf. immaculate - spotless); *adj.- macular.*

magna- large, great

mal- abnormal, bad

Malignant (MAL-ig-nant) cancerous cells which invade other body parts

Malpighian canal AKA longitudinal duct of the epoophoron

Malpighian layer AKA germinative zone of the epidermis.

Mamma: *Lt. = breast; adj.- mammary.* **(MAM-ar-ree)** a modified sweat gland in the breast that serves as the gland of milk secretion for nourishment of the young

mast- pertaining to the breast

Mastectomy removal or 1 or more breasts or parts thereof

maz- breast

meat- (mee-AYT) opening

medi- middle intermediate

Medial (MEE-dee-al) *Lt. medius = middle adj medial* a directional term describing a part lying nearer to the vertical midline of the body relative to another part.

Median: *Lt. medianus = in the middle.*

medo- to do with the penis

Medulla (meh-DUL-ah) an inner, or deeper, part of an organ. e.g. the medulla of the kys, the medulla of the adrenal gland & the LN. ≠ cortex

meg- large

megalo- very large

meio- (mĭ-oh) reduced, contraction

Meiosis (MĬ-oh-sis) germ cell division where the genetic material is halved (2n ➜ n) as a device for future fertilization (as opposed to Mitosis 2n ➜ 2n)

mel- limb, cheek

melan- black

Melanocortin a peptide H which exerts its effects by binding to the melanocortin receptors : e.g. ACTH, endorphin, lipotropin, MSH. All are derived from pro-opiomelanocortin in the pituitary gland, & play a major role in the E homeostasis.

Membrane (MEM-brayn) *Lt. membrana = a thin sheet; adj.- membranous* a thin sheet of tissue that lines or covers body structures. It may contain a thin layer of CT ± epithelium

Membranous bone a type of embryonic osseous tissue representing early skeletal development in a late embryo.

men- menses

Menarche (men-ARK-ee) *Gk: men = moon; arkhe = beginning*
the time of the first menstruation (~12 - 13yo)

Menopause (men-oh-PORZ) AKA Climacteric - when the ovaries cease to secrete Hs and so menstruation ceases. It is defined as the last menstrual period generally 4 yrs after the changes begin to occur in the H cycle & the levels of Oestrogen & Progesterone ↓ due to the failing ovary. Although there may be an abrupt cessation of periods, on average periods continue irregularly for up to 4 yrs before ceasing altogether. Average age of onset 48-52 yo. *see also Premature Ovarian Failure*

Menorrhagia excessive menstrual bleeding

Menses AKA Periods

Menstral cup cup to go over the cervix to catch the menstrual blood as an alternative to menstral pads or tampons

Menses (MEN-seez) *Lt mensis = month* **AKA Menstruation AKA Catamenia AKA Menstruum** the material discharged from the vagina during menstruation

ment- mind, chin

mer- part, segment

mes- middle

Merocrine secretions which are due to exocytosis

Mesoderm (MEEZ-oh-derm) *Gk. mesos = middle, & derma = skin*
the middle of the three primary germ layers in a developing embryo that forms the muscles, the heart and BVs, & the CT.

Mesothelium (mez-oh-THEE-lee-um) a simple squamous epithelium lining parts of the body's ventral cavity.

meta- subsequent, transformation, b/n, changing after

Metabolic syndrome AKA Syndrome X AKA Insulin-resistance syndrome is a collection of conditions that often occur together & ↑ DM2, & cardiovascular disease.
If there are more than 3 of the following in a individual then they may have metabolic syndrome

- central obesity – excess fat in & around the abdomen
- hypertension
- ↑ B [TGAs]
- ↓ B[HDLs] – the good cholesterol
- IFG ie ↑ B[glucose] but not high enough to be diagnosed as DM2.

Metrorrhagia irregular uterine bleeding often due to H imbalance (**AKA Breakthrough bleeding**) or at menopause

micro- small

Microvilli (mĭ-kroh-VIL-ee) (mv) extensions of the cm filled with cytoplasm, ↑ absorptive surface area of the cell.

mid- middle

milli- thousandth

minimus- smallest

Minor- smaller of 2 things e.g. Psoas Minor m lies deep & is smaller than Psoas Major m *see also Major*

mio- reduced contraction

Mitosis (MĬ-toh-sis) - normal cell division where the genetic material is unchanged b/n the mother & daughter cells

mnem- (mem) memory

Molecule a neutral group of atoms held together by ionic or covalent bonds - however it is often also a term used for a charged polyatomic group which are technically *Radicals*

Monomers individual units of a larger structure - usually with the building up of extracellular fibres e.g. collagen *see also polymers*

Monocyte (MON-oh-sĭt) a large, agranular WBC that is phagocytic. If the cell moves from the BS to the ECT, it is called a mØ.

morph- (morf) shape

Morphology: *Gk. morphos = form, & logos = word or relation*; hence, study of pattern of structure; *adj. morphological.*

Mucosa (MEW-koh-zuh) T in the GIT beneath the epithelial lining

multi- many

myc- (mĭs-) fungal

myel- RBM, SC

myo- (mĭ-oh) muscle

Myocardium (mĭ-oh-KAHR-dee-um) *Gk. mys = muscle, & kardia = heart, adj. myocardial.* the primary layer of the heart wall, composed of cardiac muscle T.

Myometrium (mĭ-oh-MEE-tree-um) the SM layer in the wall of the uterus.

Myotome: *Gk. mys = muscle, & tome = a cutting*; a group of muscles innervated by spinal segment.

myx- (mix) mucoid

Myxoedema AS myxedema (MIX-e-deem-uh) - swelling under the skin due to hypothyroidism – hard oedema (mucoid) in the subcutaneous Ts

N

narc- stupor

necro- (NEK-roh) death

Necrosis (ne-KROH-sis) death of a cell, a group of cells, or a tissue due to disease.

Negation processes which render a male impotent

neo- (NEE-oh) new

Neonatal: *adj.Gk. neos = new & Lt. natos = born*; hence, new-born.

Neoplasm (NEE-OH-plasm) any abnormal growth of T or proliferation of cells not under physiological control – may be benign or malignant

nephro- (NEF-rho) renal kidney

neur- nerve

Neuroendocrine axis the structural & functional basis for interactions b/n the Brain, Hs, & glands to complex stimuli such as stress or reproduction. It refers to any of these 3 pathways & their feedback mechanisms.

Neuron (N) (NEW-ron) *Gk. neuron = nerve adj. neurium.* **AKA Nerve cell** *adj. neural* a cell of NT characterized by its specialization to conduct impulses (conductivity).

Neuropeptide short chain PPs compounds which act as neurotransmitters

neutro- neutral

noci- (noh-SEE) pain

Nubility the state of being fertile- i.e. regular continual ovulation

Nuclear membrane (nm) the double bilipid incomplete membrane which separates the nuclear material from the cytoplasm. It is often continuous with some internal cellular membranes e.g. ER, GA & vacuoles

Nucleolus (NEW-klee-oh-lus) little nucleus - a small unbound collection of RNA w/in the nucleus which varies in size, shape & presence due to the activity of the cell. It is the site of rRNA synthesis & dispersement, & the assembly of ribosomes. It appears as a darkly staining spot(s) in the nucleus *pl nucleoli*

Nucleophile *"nucleus loving", or "positive-charge loving"* - a chemical species that donates an electron pair to form a covalent bond, generally a strong base

Nucleosome a coil of DNA wrapped around a histone core as a form of organized packing

Nucleus (NEW-klee-us) *Lt. = kernel or nut.* It contains the genetic material to determine protein structure & function, the DNA. It is enveloped by a double-layered mem.

null- none

O

ob- against, in front of

oedem- (er-DEEM-) swelling (AS edem-)

-oid like

olig- scant deficient few little

Oligomennorrhoea minimal menstrual bleeding < 20mls

-ology (o-loh-jee) study of

-oma tumor or lump

Oöcyte (OH-oh-sït) AKA Ovum, egg a gamete produced w/n an ovary.

or- ora- Lt. ora = margin or edge **mouth**

Oöphorectomy surgical removal of the ovaries

Orexigenic (OR-ex-ee-jen-ik) - appetite stimulating - can be from Hs, medications &/or other substances e.g. Hs with an orexigenic SE which includes: most steroid Hs, cannabinoids, seretonin, anti DM2 drugs, INS, sugar & fructose (≠ **anorexic**)

Organ a group of Ts & cells which are bound together to perform a specific function

Organelle (or-gan-EL) a component of a cell that has a consistent, similar structure in other cells & performs a particular function

Orgasm intense paroxysmal emotional excitement, the climax of SA towards the end of coitus usually accompanied by ejaculation in the male, associated with a sudden ↑ Oxytocin & Prolactin

-osis condition of / disease of – non-inflammatory

osteo (os-TEE-oh) pertaining to bone

Osteoporosis (OP) *bone poverty* significant loss of bone, including loss of bone trabeculae **(t)**. This is not reversible & leads to pathological fractures **(f)**, at points of great stress: the hip & VC are common sites. The incidence of OP ↑ after menopause, due in part to the ↓ oestrogen levels, *see also Menopause, Oestrogen & OPG.*

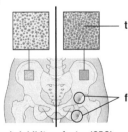

Osteoprotegerin AKA osteoclastogenesis inhibitory factor (OPG) is a glycoprotein (401 AAs) & a member of the TNF-receptor family. It acts as a decoy receptor for RANKL. By binding RANKL, it prevents RANKL binding with osteoblasts & forming osteoclasts, & ↑ bone resorption. OPG is stimulated by the oestrogen. As oestrogen ↓ after menopause bone resorption ↑. This may lead to OP. *see also Menopause*

-osteum (os-tee-um) pertaining to bone

Ovary (OH-vahr-ee) *Lt. ovum = egg pl* - ova the female gonad, or primary reproductive organ that produces gametes & female sex Hs

Ovulation the release of the oöcyte from the ovary from a mature follicle

Ovum AKA Öocyte AKA Egg *pl ova*

oxy- (OKS-ee) sharp

P

pali- recurrence

pan- general overall

par- beside

para- against aside abnormal unequal

Parenchyma (pa-REN-kïm-ah) *Gk para = beside or near, en = in & chein = to pour* the functioning elements of an organ as opposed to the structural or supporting elements (≠ stroma)

Parietal (pa-RÏ-eh-tal) *Lt. parietalis, pertaining to paries = wall* pertaining to the outer wall of a cavity or organ i.e. parietal layer of the pericardium outer of the 2 layers of the pericardium (≠ visceral).

Pars: *Lt. = part.*

path-/ -pathy disease / disease of

Pathogenesis – origin or cause of a disease

-penia (PEEN-ee-uh) lack of

per- through, excessive

peri- around, about, beyond

Perilipin AKA lipid droplet-associated protein (PLIN) a protein covering the surface of mature lipid droplets in adipocytes, & restricting access to lipases so that fat is not randomly hydrolysed. Phosphorylation of perilipin allows fats to rise to the surface of the droplet & so access lipases for hydrolysis.

Perimenopause the period b/n the cessation of the periods for a year (the menopause) & the onset of hormonal symptoms, which may be up to 3 yrs long & may extend into the menopause

Peristalsis: *Gk. peri = around & stellein - to constrict*; a circular constriction passing as a wave along a muscular tube; *adj.-* peristaltic.

Peritoneum (per-it-on-NEE-um) *Gk. periteino = to stretch around* the extensive serous membrane associated with the abdominopelvic cavity. *adj.-* peritoneal.

pero- stunted, malformed

Peroxisome vesicles .2-0.5μm containing dense particle involved in the catabolism of FAs & the synthesis of plasma proteins & cholesterol, they contain relevant enzymes to help in this process & are commonest in hepatocytes and only have a monolipid layer - different from most ic mem bound vesicles, which have bilipid layers

phago (FAY-goh) to eat

Phagocytosis the active ingestion & digestion of larger particles w/n a cell

Pheromone (FER-oh-mohn) *Gk phero = to transport; hormone = to stimulate* is a secreted or excreted chemical factor which acts outside the body to cause a behavioural change in the receiver. Examples of these are: *alarm pheromones; food pheromones & sex pheromones.*

Phosphorylation - addition of 1 or more phosphate radicals to a structure - usually protein, often to ↑ hydrophilia

physi- (FIZ-ee) natural

Plasma is blood w/o its cellular components see also Serum

plan- flat level, to wander

-plasia (FAY-zee-uh) growth

Plasma membrane AKA cell membrane (cm)

plat- broad flat

pleo- (PLEE-oh) many

pleur- (PLER) lungs respiratory

Pleura (PLEW-rah) *Gk. = a rib* but has not come to mean the serous membrane lining the lungs (visceral layer) & inner rib & intercostal surfaces (parietal layer) assoc. with the lungs

Plexus (PLEKS-uhs) *Lt. = a network or plait.* a network of interconnecting Ns, veins, or lymphatic vessels

pluri- several

poikilo- (POYK-il-oh)irregular

polio- (POH-lee-oh) grey

poly- (POL-ee) many

Polypeptide cells AKA γ gamma cells of Pancreas

por- passageway

postero- posterior part

Posterior (pos-TEE-ree-or) *Lt. post = behind (in place or time).* a directional term describing the location of a part being toward the back or rear side relative to another part.

Posterior pituitary gland AKA Neurohypophysis the part of the pituitary gland at the base of the brain consisting of the axons of Ns originating in the hypothalamus & supporting T

Postpartum thyrotoxicosis *see Hashimoto thyrotoxicosis*

prae- in front of, before

pre- in front of before

Premature ovarian failure shutdown or failure of the ovarian function < 40yo occurs in 1% of females. Aetiologies - autoimmune, genetic

Premenstrual syndrome syndrome of tenseness & irritability prior to the menstral bleeding

Pretibial myxoedema AS myxedema sign of hypothyroidism caused by excessive laying down of mucopolysaccharides (AKA glycosaminoglycans) e.g. hyaluronic acid & chondroitin sulphate in the skin rendering it thickened and inelastic

Prepuce: *Lt. praeputium = foreskin* of penis or clitoris.

presby- old

prim- first

Primary germ layer one of 3 layers of cells that differentiate during the embryonic stage to give rise to all tissues in the body. They are the endoderm, mesoderm & ectoderm.

pro- in front of

Pro-inflammatory (pro-If) causing the up-regulation of inflammatory mediators

Prognosis (prog-NOH-sis) *Gk pro- = in front of & gno- = to know – fore knowledge* hence the expected outcome of a disease

Prolapse (PROH-laps) to slip & fall out of place

Proptosis (PROH-toh-sis) bulging yes - generally due to lid retraction, & pressure at the back fo the eye causing it to move forward (≠ Ptosis) see thyroid eye disease (TED)

Prostate (PROS-stayt) gland *Gk. pro = before, & Lt. = statum = stood* something which stands before – e.g.the prostate gland stands before the urinary bladder. A walnut-shaped gland surrounding the urethra as it emerges from the urinary bladder in males. Its secretions contribute to semen.

Protein a series of > 50 AAs bound together with peptide bonds. May be branched, highly folded & made up of many peptide subunits. A protein is generally larger & more complex than a PP, but there is an overlap in these terms. *see also AAs, peptide bonds, & PPs*

Proximal (PROKS-i-mal) *Lt. proxime = nearest* a directional term indicating a body part that is located nearer to the origin or point of attachment to the trunk than another; opposite of distal

pseudo- (syoo-doh) false

Ptosis (TOH-sis) drooping eyelid, in severe conditions the visual field os affected by the presence f the eyelid over the pupil (≠ Proptosis)

Pubarche (pew-BARK-ee) the first appearance of pubic hairs (~10 - 13yo), often slightly earlier in the female, due to the ↑ androgens from the adrenal cortex &/or testes

Puberty: *Lt. puber = adult*; hence, the time when hair appears in the pubic region - i.e., near the pubis - as a secondary sexual characteristic. Maturation of an immature non-fertile body to a fertile body under H influence

pyelo- basin , pelvis (generally renal pelvis)

pykno- (PIK-noh) thick, dense

pyo- (PI-oh) pus

R

Radicals charged atomic particles or charged polyatomic groups which may be bound to larger molecules or freely disassociated and "unbound" - *free radicals* - refer to unbound charged ions or molecules - which are highly reactive

RANK/RANKL osteoclast surface receptor / receptor activator of nuclear factor-kappaB ligand proteins which together activate & ↑ the formation of osteoclasts & so ↑ bone resorption.

re- return, back again

Recommended dietary intake AKA recommended daily allowance (RDA) the recommended levels of consumption of essential food substance generally determined by the regulatory body of the country, in Australia this is the TGA - Therapeutic Goods Administration

ren- (REEN) kidney

Rete (REE-tee): *Lt. = a net; adj. reticular:* hence, a network of veins or tubules.

retro- prefix *Lt. = backwards.* located behind

rhe- flow

rheum- (ROOM) mucoid or watery discharge / relating to joint pain

rhod- red

rigor- *Lt rigor = stiffness*

S

schiz- split

Secosteroid (sek-OH-ster-OID): *Lt secare = to cut; stere = solid 3 dimensional* a subclass of steroid with a break in the carbon ring, e.g.C9-10 secosteroid e.g. cholecalciterol (Vita D3)

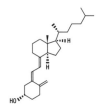

Secrete: (se-KREET) *Lt. secretus = separated*; hence, to produce a chemical substance by glandular activity *adj. secretory; noun, secretion.*

Semen: *Lt. = seed; adj. seminal* (seminal vesicle).

semi- half partial

Senescence signs associated with aging e.g. in a cell the accumulation of lipofuscin is related to age

seps- decay

Sex hormone-binding globulin (SHBG) AKA sex steroid-binding globulin (SSBG) is a glycoprotein that binds to the steroid Hs, sex Hs & cortisol & other corticosteroids. One of these is transcortin.

Soma (SOH-ma) *Gk. = the body adj. somatic* pertaining to the body or the main part of an organ or a cell but not the viscera

Somite: *Gk. soma = body*, hence an embryonic body segment.

spir- coiled, respiration, breath

stas- stopped

-statin - stopping

steat- (STEE-at) fat

steno- narrow

Stenosis (STEN-oh-sis) *Gk = narrowing* hence narrowing of a duct, BV or other passage

Stigma the area on the ovarian surface **(1)** where the Graäfian follicle will burst at ovulation. It is composed of the BM of the follicle **(4)** + the ovarian BM under the germinal epithelium **(2)**. With maturation the area b/n the follicle & ovarian surface thins, pushing aside the internal layers of the tunica albuginea **(3)** & theca interna & externa **(5)** of the stroma of the ovary & weakens

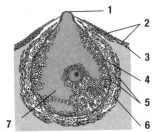

due to LH & local cytokines. The stigma ruptures at ovulation, with ⬆ P from SM **(6)** contraction, releasing the oöcyte **(8)** + follicular fluid **(7)**. The stigma heals with the transformation of the follicle into the CL.

Stoma: *Gk. = a mouth.*

Stratum *Lt. = a covering sheet,* or layer. generally referring to the skin layers pertaining to a multiple-layered arrangement *adj. - stratified*

Striae AKA Stretch marks (STRI-ee) common acquired condition, due to H changes & physical stress on the skin. They present as parallel bands of discoloration on the skin, assoc. with growth spurts or rapid weight gain, as in pregnancy. Initially bright red or deep purple, they gradually fade to atrophic white bands, which are permanent. They thin & weaken: the epidermis (E),⬇ the depth & number of dermal papillae (P) & they place the collagen closer to the surface (Sc), forming a separation b/n the skin with dermal papillae & the thinner stretched striae (S), *sing. stria* **(STRI-uh)**.

Striae Gravidarum – stretch marks of pregnancy often with a single midline striae Linea Nigra (LN)

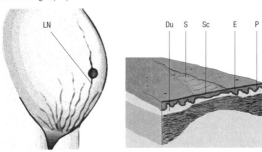

Stroma (STROH-mah) *Gk. = bed or mattress supporting bed of cells,* CT or matrix upon which the parenchyma builds

sub- under less than partial

sud- sweat

Sudoriferous (syoo'-dor-IF-er-us) gland AKA sweat gland an exocrine gland located in the skin that secretes sweat.

Sudomotor: *Lt. sudor = sweat, and movere = to move,* hence stimulate the sweat glands.

suf- under

super- over

Superficial (soo-per-FISH-al) *Lt. super = above & facies = surface;* hence, nearer the body surface (≠ deep).

Superior (soo-PEER-ee-or) AKA Craniad AKA Cephalad *Lt. superus = above* a directional term indicating the location of a part that is nearer to the head region than another.

supra- *Lt. prefix = superior to* **above over**

sym- together union association

Symporter AS Simporter a cm **(1)** protein transporter **(2)** which moves 2 or more molecules or ions **(3)** simultaneously in the same direction **(B)** a type of co-transporter (also antiporter - which transports 2 or molecules in opposite directions - c.f. exchange transportation **(C)** or a uniporter **(A)** which can only move 1 substance at a time.

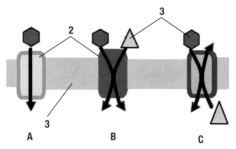

A   **B**   **C**

Synapse (sïn-APS) *Gk. syn = with, & aptein = to join* the join b/n the axon of one N & the dendrite or cell body of another N; the zone of the passage of the impulse from one N to another

Syncytium: *Gk. syn = with & kytos = cell,* a multinucleate mass of protoplasm formed by cells merging c.f. Giant cells & the outer syncytium of the placenta

Syndrome: *Gk. syn = with, & dromos = running;* i.e. a group of SS, characteristic of a certain pathology.

T

tect- covering

Testis (TEHS-tihs) AKA Testicle: *Lt. testiculus = the male gonad. Lt. testis = a witness. pl. - testes* one of a pair of male gonads (sex glands) located w/n the scrotum that produces sperm cells & testosterone. Under Roman law, no man could bear witness (*testify*) unless he possessed both testes.

Testosterone a steroidal H secreted by interstitial cells (cells of Leydig) located w/n the testes. It promotes the development of ♂ 2° sex characteristics & the development of spermatozoa. It peaks at 18yo in most males ↓ @ 1% per year. If there is a sudden larger ↓ there may be symptoms see also Andropause

terti (ter-shi-) third

Tetrahydrobiopterin (TET-RU-hi-droh-bi-oh-tair-in) is a cofactor used with the **aromatic AA hydroxylase** enzymes; the first step in the synthesis of the catecholamines, melatonin & serotonin. It is also a cofactor in the reaction for the production of NO by the **nitric oxide synthases**.

Theca: *Gk. theka = a capsule, sheath.*

Thelarche (thel-ARK-ee) *Gk: thele = nipple; arkhe = beginning* secondary breast development, generally in girls associated with menarche, but generally preceding it (~8yo). Breasts develop under the influence of oestradial, & this occurs in young males as well - termed gynaecomastia. *see also Menarche*

Thrombus a blood clot that has formed & is attached to a vein or artery.

Thyroid: *Gk. thyreos = shield, & eidos = shape or form*; shaped like a shield (shields the glottis).

Tissue (T) (TI-shoo) a group of similar cells that combine to form a common function.

Totipotent refers to a cell which is truly able to transform itself into any other cell - used to be thought that this was only the germ cells of the body - but it is now possible to transform many of the other cells in the body to this form - *stem cells*

trans- crossing changing

Transcortin a sex H binding globulin

Trauma (TRAW-mah) *Gk injury*, wound physical or psychological

tri- three

trop- (TROHP) turn change

troph- (TROHF) nutrition

Tumor AS Tumour: (TEW-mah) *Lt. tumere = to swell* indicating an IF process (fluid swelling) or a neoplasm when the swelling is from new cellular growth

Tunica (TEW-nik-uh): *Lt. = shirt*; hence a covering, generally referring to layers around an organ or T.

U

uni- first one

Uterus: (YEW-tehr-uhs) *Lt. = womb.* a hollow muscular organ in the ♀ reproductive system that serves as a site of embryo implantation, development & menstruation.

Utricle: diminutive of *Lt. uterus = womb.*

Urinary bladder (yew-rin-AR-ee BLAD-ar) AKA Bladder a hollow muscular organ located at the floor of the pelvic cavity that temporarily stores urine.

V

Vagina (vaj-Ĭ-nuh) *Lt. = sheath; hence, invagination is the acquisition of a sheath by pushing inwards into a membrane,* a tubular, muscular organ of the female reproductive system extending b/n the vulva & the uterus & *evagination is similar but produced by pushing outwards. adj. vaginal*

Vaginal Discharge is any fluid / material oozing from the vagina - normal may be clear, white , yellow ± white flecks & may ↑ mid-cycle & become ↓ viscous. The pH is generally acidic (~4.3) which prevents Ins in the vagina. Any changes may indicate infection in this area

vaso- pertaining to BF

Vasomotor instability BVs in particular skin arterioles become unstable & allow for a sudden ↑ in the dermal BF, causing flushing & heat - generally the cause of hot flushes experienced in menopause & its assoc. H changes

Vascular (VAS-kyew-lar) *Lt. vasculum, diminutive of vas;* hence, pertaining or containing BVs.

ven- vein

vesic- to do with the bladder

Vesica: *Lt. = bladder, adj.- vesical.*

Vesicle (VEEZ-i-kel) *diminutive of Lt. vesica = bladder, hence a little bladder* a small sac containing a fluid. In the cell, it is a membranous sac w/n the cytoplasm which contains cellular products or waste materials, & creates a microenvironment w/n the cell *(see also organelle)* .

Vesicula: diminutive of *Lt. vesica = bladder; seminal vesicle.*

Visceral (VIHS-er-ahl) *Lt. viscus = an internal organ* pertaining to the internal components (mainly the organs) of a body cavity; pertaining to the outer surface of an internal organ ≠ parietal.

Viscus: *Lt. = an internal organ, pl. - viscera, adj.- visceral.*

Vital: *Lt. vita = life.*

Vitelline: *Lt. vitellus = yolk.*

Vitreous: *Lt. vitreus = glassy.*

vivi- alive

volv- turn

Vulgar: *Lt vulgaris = usual*; common, plentiful

Womb AKA Uterus

xanth- (ZANTH) yellow

xeno- (ZEN-oh) different

xenohormones H-like substances derived from synthetic or natural substances which imitate the actions of Hs & may disrupt normal endocrine processes e.g. xenoestrogens, which can have a H disruptive effect on puberty. These substances do not necessarily have similar structures to the H they affect.

xero- (ZAIR-roh) dry

Z

Zona (ZOH-nah) *Lt. = a belt; hence, a circular band* an area smaller than a region in an organ as in the adrenal gland

Zonule: diminutive of zona.

zyg- yoke

-zyme (-ZĬM) enzyme

Amino Acids (AAs) - general

generic formula of AA linear
generic formula of AA splayed
2D structure of AA

AAs are the building blocks of proteins, which are generally > 50 AAs. Small proteins are called polypeptides (PPs), but there is an overlap in these terms. There are 20 proteinogenic AAs found in the human. **9 essential** which must be obtained by diet & **11 non essential** which the body can synthesize.

Their structure consists of a backbone of:

AMINO group (NH_2) + α-Carbon (C) + CARBOXYLIC ACID group (COOH).

The α-C then binds an Hydrogen & a variable side chain (**R**), with its 2 remaining covalent bonds.

The molecule is asymmetrical, having 4 different structures bound to the α-C (chilarity).

It is possible to have 2 isomers of this structure, but proteins contain only the **dextrorotatory (L)** version. Hence they are **L-α-chiral AAs***.

1 **carboxyl group**
2 **amine group**
3 **α - Carbon with bound hydrogen**
4 **R side chain - varies with each AA**

* glycine & proline are exceptions

H₂NCHRCOOH

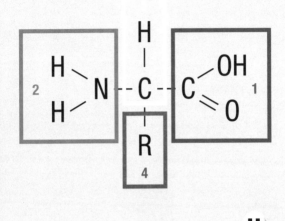

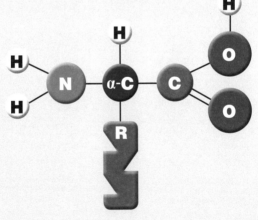

59

Amino Acids (AAs) - general

3D structure of AA
3D structure of AA - showing electrons
Zwitterion formula
Zwitterion 3D

Changing pH levels change the balance & ionization of the AA via their 2 weak acid grps (carboxyl > amino), but at most physiological pH levels ~7.4, AAs exist mainly as **Zwitterions**, having a total charge of zero the -ve charge of the carboxyl grp balanced by the +ve amine charge, but the exact isoelectric point (pI) when there is no charge at all is determined by the **R-side chain**.

The R-side chain determines most of the properties of any AA. If R is hydrophilic, the AA is described as hydrophilic etc.

Hydrophilic AAs interact with the aqueous environment & exterior surfaces of the proteins; they are involved in the formation of H-bonds & in the reactive centres of enzymes / Hs or their receptors.

Hydrophobic AAs reside predominantly in the interior of proteins, protected from the aqueous environment by hydrophilic molecules. This class of AA does not ionize nor participate in the formation of H-bonds.

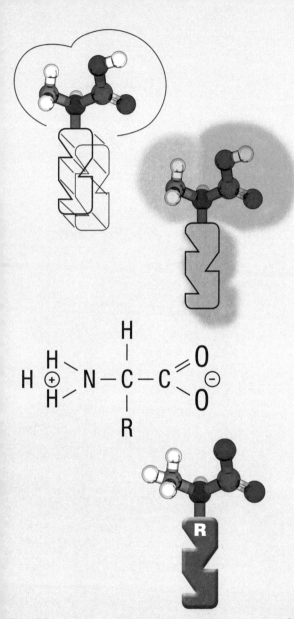

$$H \underset{H}{\overset{H}{\oplus}} N - \underset{R}{\overset{H}{C}} - C \overset{O}{\underset{O}{\diagdown}} \ominus$$

61

Amino Acids (AAs) - general

formation of a PEPTIDE bond

AAs must join together to form proteins or PPs. They do this via PEPTIDE bonds, which bind the amine (NH$_2$) & α-C together liberating water (H$_2$O), The smallest peptide is a dipeptide

5 **AA1**

6 **AA2**

7 **dipeptide**
   p = peptide bond

8 **water - H$_2$O**

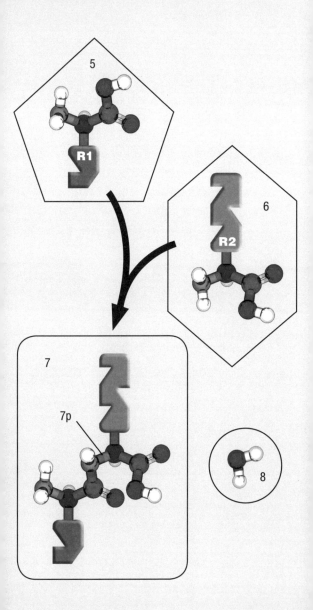

5

R1

6

R2

7

7p

8

Amino Acids - Alanine (A-Ala)

2-Aminopropanoic acid

$$CH_3 - CH - COOH$$
$$| $$
$$NH_2$$

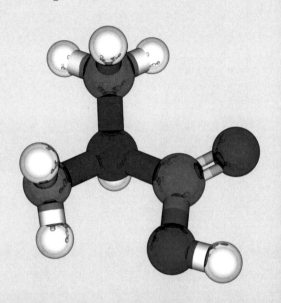

Type	Properties		Sources
aliphatic hydrophobic non polar	small MW = 71.09 pI - 6.0	non -essential from pyruvate & branched AAs glucogenic	**animal**: meat, dairy products, eggs, fish, **veg**: beans, nuts, seeds, soy, legumes, whole grains
		↑ BP ↑ E ↑ cholesterol	

© A. L. Neill

Amino Acids - Arginine (R - Arg)

2-amino-5-guanidinopentoic acid

$$HN - CH_2 - CH_2 - CH_2 - CH - COOH$$

$$\underset{\underset{NH_2}{|}}{C} = NH \qquad\qquad\qquad NH_2$$

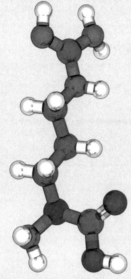

Type	Properties		Sources
aliphatic basic hydrophilic polar	+ve charge MW = 156.2 PK R grp = 12.5 pI = 5.7	semi essential from citrulline, glutamate & proline glucogenic	**animal**: meat dairy prods **plant**: wheat germ nuts & seeds
		↑ cell division ↑ healing ↑ GH ↓ BP ↓ tooth sensitivity	one of the commonest AAs

Amino Acids - Asparagine (N - Asn)

2-Amino-3-carbamoylpropanoic acid

$$H_2N - \underset{\underset{O}{\overset{\|}{}}}{C} - CH_2 - \underset{\underset{NH_2}{|}}{CH} - COOH$$

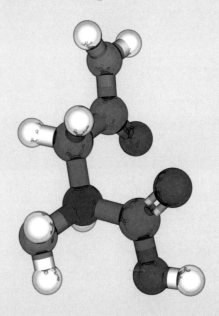

Type	Properties		Sources
branched acidic amide hydrophilic polar	-ve charge MW = 115.2 pK R grp = 3.9	non-essential from oxaloacetate glucogenic	**animal**: dairy, meat eggs & fish **plant**: asparagus, sprouting vegs potatoes legumes artificial sweetener similar to Aspartate, Glutamate Glutamine swap amide grps may substitute for them
		helps in brain dev	produces ammonia

Amino Acids - Aspartic acid / Aspartate (D - Asp)

2-Aminobutanedioic acid

$$HOOC - CH_2 - CH - COOH$$
$$| $$
$$NH_2$$

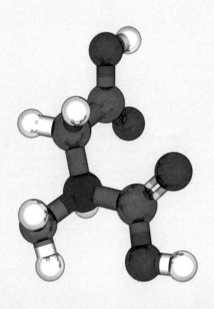

Type	Properties		Sources
acidic hydrophilic polar	- ve charge MW = 115.2 pK R grp = 3.9	non-essential from oxaloacetate glucogenic	**animal**: oysters, **plant**: asparagus, sprouting vgs artificial sweetener similar to Asparagine, Glutamate, Glutamine swap amide grps may substitute for them
		fixes metal ions weak neurotransmitter	

Amino Acids - Cysteine (C - Cys)

2 amino-3-sulphuhydrylpropanoic acid

$$HS - CH_2 - CH - COOH$$
$$NH_2$$

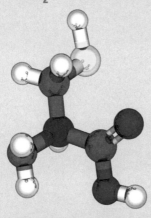

Type	Properties		Sources
nucleophilic hydrophobic polar via the **thiol grp (-SH)**	**disulphide bonds (S-S)** contribute to the active centres of proteins & recep e.g. insulin recep stabilizes, bends proteins MW = 121.1 pK R group = 8.3 pI - 5.1	semi-essential from serine & methionine only absorbed as cystine glucogenic	**animal**: pork poultry, hair **plant**: peppers onions garlic green veg
Cysteine-SH + HS-Cysteine <—> Cysteine-S-S-Cysteine = CYSTINE H_2N HO O S S O OH NH_2	↑ hair gth ↑ wool grth ↑ antioxidant ↑ expectorant cig additive food additive E920 food flavouring hair perm solutions		contribs to protein conformation forms stable proteins used in the GIT (harsh conditions) similar to Methionine

© A. L. Neill

Amino Acids - Glutamic acid / Glutamate (E - Glu)

2-Aminopentanedioic acid

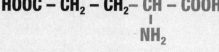

HOOC – CH$_2$ – CH$_2$ – CH – COOH
|
NH$_2$

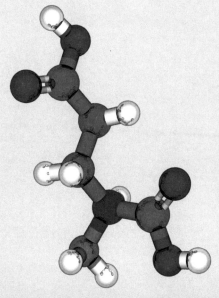

Type	Properties		Sources
aliphatic acidic hydrophilic polar	-ve charge MW = 146.2 pK R grp = 4.1 pI = 5.7	non-essential glucogenic most abundant excitatory neurotransmitter + precursor of GABA	**abundant in most foods** similar to Asparagine, Aspartate, Glutamine swap amide grps may substitute for them
	↑ learning ↑ memory	food flavourings (monosodium glutamate)	excitotoxicity in excess (from neural damage liberates large amounts in the brain) ↑ fits ↑ strokes

Amino Acids - Glutamine (Q - Gln)

2-Amino-4-carbamoylbutanoic acid

$$H_2N - \underset{\underset{O}{\parallel}}{C} - CH_2 - CH_2 - \underset{\underset{NH_2}{\mid}}{CH} - COOH$$

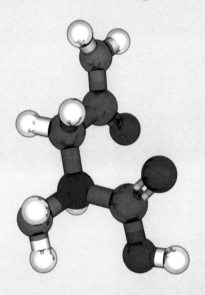

Type	Properties		Sources
amide acid hydrophilic polar	no charge MW = 146.2 pI = 5.7	non-essential *but the body needs large amounts* from oxaloacetate glucogenic	**abundant in most foods most abundant AA in nature and the body** similar to Aspartate, Asparagine Glutamate swap amide grps may substitute for them
	strong neurotransmitter Xs the BBB directly	store for ammonia E source nitrogen source	

Amino Acids - Glycine (G - Gly)

aminoethanoic acid AKA aminoacetic acid

$$H - CH - COOH$$
$$\quad\quad NH_2$$

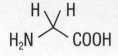

SYMMETRICAL
NON CHIRAL

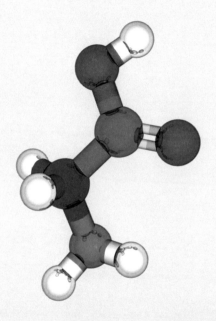

Type	Properties		Sources
hydrophobic + hydrophilic = amphoteric polar	small - flexible MW = 57.05 pl = 5.97	non-essential derived from serine glucogenic	**abundant in most foods** **artificial sweeteners drug excipient/ facilitator**
	not chiral / R = H	↑ collagen synthesis CNS inhibitory neurotransmitter	↑ sleep ↓ schizophrenia

Amino Acids - Histidine (H - His)

2-Amino-4-carbamoylbutanoic acid

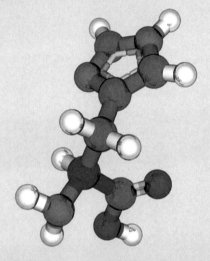

Type	Properties		Sources
imidazole ring can donate or accept a proton - shuttles protons - back & forth basic hydrophilic polar	+ve charge MW = 137.2 PK R grp = 6.0	essential glucogenic	not a great deal needed small requirements **animal:** fish eggs meat **plant:** cereal grains
	↑ IR ↑ IfR	in the reactive centre of regulatory enzymes, partic metalo-proteins eg haemoglobin used as a proton shuttle binds metal cations	

Amino Acids - Isoleucine (I - Ile)

2-Amino-3-methylpentanoic acid

H₃C – H₂C
H₃C
CH – CH – COOH
NH₂

CHIRAL SIDE CHAIN

$$H_3C-H_2C-CH-CH-COOH$$

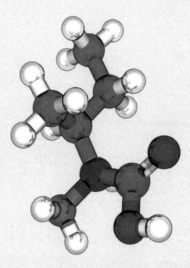

Type	Properties		Sources
branched hydrophobic non polar	MW - 131.2 pI - 6.0	essential glucogenc & ketogenic	**animal sources:** most meats have large quantities it is found readily in diet **plants:** soy beans similar to Leucine, Valine
	forms sterols in muscles & AT ↑ muscle grth	requires Biotin (Vita B7) to be catabolised w/o this metabolic disorders of muscles cognition etc develop	

Amino Acids - Leucine (L - Leu)

2-Amino-3-methylpentanoic acid

$$H_3C$$
$$H_3C$$ $$CH - CH_2 - CH - COOH$$
$$NH_2$$

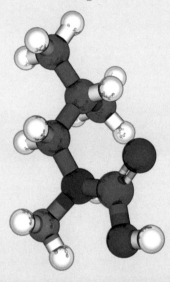

Type	Properties		Sources
branched hydrophobic non polar	MW - 131.2 pI 5.98	essential ketogenic	**animal:** fish , pork chicken & egg **plant:** soy, nuts, wheat germ
	major component of buffer proteins - eg ferritin forms sterols in muscles & AT ↑↑ muscle grth	requires Biotin (Vita B7) to be catabolised w/o this metabolic disorders of muscles cognition etc develop	toxicity causes acute: delirium long term: pellagra (diarrhoea, dermatitis, dementia , death) related to Isoleucine, Valine

Amino Acids - Lysine (K - Lys)

2,6-Diaminohexanoic acid; 2,6-Diammoniohexanoic acid

$$H_2N - (CH_2)_4 - CH - COOH$$
$$\qquad\qquad\qquad\quad |$$
$$\qquad\qquad\qquad\; NH_2$$

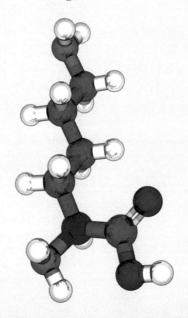

Type	Properties		Sources
aliphatic basic hydrophilic polar	+ve charge MW = 128.2 PK R grp = 10.8	essential ketogenic	**animal:** red meat, fish **plant:** sprouting seeds, often the least AA in grains *increasing lysine content increases the quality of a grain*
	needed to form X-links in elastin & collagen	involved in intracellular secretion ➜ ER GA & lysosomes	**may protect against Herpes outbreaks** ↓ **anxiety via serotonin** similar to Arginine

Amino Acids - Methionine (M - Met)

2-amino-4-(methylthio) butanoic acid

$$H_3C - S - (CH_2)_2 - CH - COOH$$
$$\underset{NH_2}{|}$$

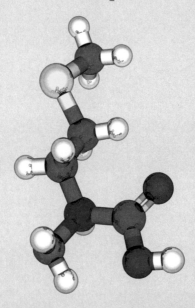

Type	Properties		Sources
aliphatic hydrophobic non polar	MW = 149.2 pl - 5.7	essential glucogenic	**animal:** egg **plant:** sesame seeds, nuts similar to Cysteine
	↓ lifespan ↓ aging ↑ grey hair ↑ urine acidity	belongs to aspartate family	used in protein synthesis & methylation

Amino Acids - Phenylanaline (F - Phe)

2-Amino-3-phenylpropanoic acid

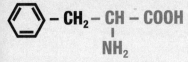

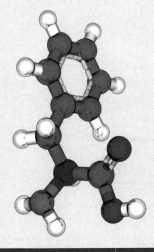

Type	Properties		Sources
aromatic - ability to absorb UV light naturally fluorescent	no charge MW = 147.2	essential converts to Tyrosine glucogenic & ketogenic	**animal:** breast milk, dairy
			plant: soy, seeds & nuts
			artificial sweetener
			similar to Trytophan, Tyrosine must be actively transported aX the BBB
hydrophobic non polar			
	↑ analgesic ↑ antidepressant	Phenyl-Ketonurics cannot metabolise this AA & its build up causes severe abnormalities	precursor of neurotransmitters noradrenalin & dopamine

Amino Acids - Proline (P - Pro) IMINO acid

Pyrrolidine-2-carboxylic acid

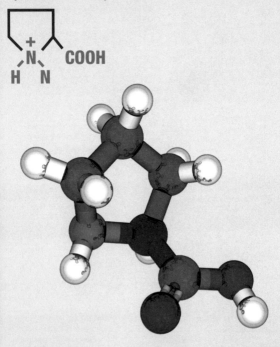

Type	Properties		Sources
imino - amide grp binds back to the α-C-forms an inflexible ring hydrophobic non polar (but may be on the outer of proteins)	no charge MW = 115.1	non essential from glutamic acid glucogenic	**animal:** egg common in most foods
	forces protein shape changes	↓ collagen ↓ CT integrity tone ↓ muscle strength ↓ aging hydroxyproline needs Vita C	

Amino Acids - Serine (S - Ser)

2-Amino-3-hydroxypropanoic acid

$$HO - CH_2 - CH - COOH$$
$$|$$
$$NH_2$$

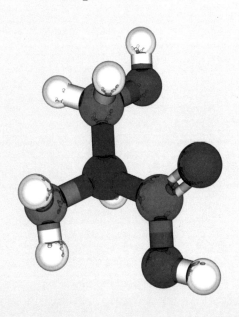

Type	Properties		Sources
nucleophilic hydroxyl groups hydrophilic polar	MW = 105.1 pK R group = 13 pI - 6.0	non -essential glucogenic	**abundant in the diet plants mainly - soy** similar to Threonine
	↑ IR ↑ IfR	↑ biosynthesis of purines & pyrimidines (DNA & RNA bases) sphingolipids & folate C donor in protein synthesis	component of cm precursor of many AAs

Amino Acids - Threonine (T-Thr)

2-Amino-3-hydroxybutanoic acid

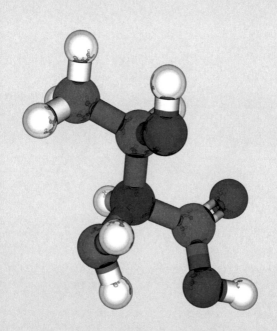

Type	Properties		Sources
nucleophilic non-aromatic with hydroxyl groups hydrophilic polar	MW = 119.1 pK Rgroup = 13 pI - 5.6	essential glucogenic & ketogenic	**animal:** cheese, fish **plant:** soy, sesame seeds, green vegs similar to Serine

Amino Acids - Trytophan (W - Trp)

2-Amino-3-(1H-indol-3-yl)propanoic acid

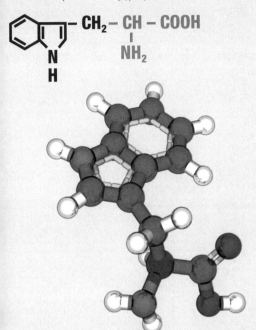

Type	Properties		Sources
aromatic - ability to absorb UV light naturally fluorescent + an indole grp hydrophobic non polar	no charge MW = 204.2 pI - 5.9	essential glucogenic & ketogenic	**animal:** dairy products, eggs **plant:** soy, seeds rice, fruit other : chocolate similar to Phenylalanine, Tyrosine
	↑ sleep pattern ↑ memory ↓ cholesterol ↓ depression ↓ anxiety	precursor to Serotonin / Melatonin / Niacin	must be actively transported aX the BBB

Amino Acids - Tyrosine (Y - Tyr)

L-2-Amino-3-(4-hydroxyphenyl)propanoic acid

$$HO - \langle\rangle - CH_2 - CH - COOH$$
$$| \\ NH_2$$

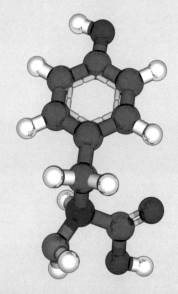

Type	Properties		Sources
aromatic - ability to absorb UV light naturally fluorescent hydrophobic polar	no charge MW = 181.2 pK R grp = 10.1	semi-essential from Phenylalanine glucogenic & ketogenic	**animal:** breast milk, dairy **plant:** seeds & nuts similar to Phenylalanine
		precursor to melanin (skin pigment) / adrenalin / noradrenalin thyroid Hs	

Amino Acids - Valine (V - Val)

2-amino-3-methylbutanoic acid

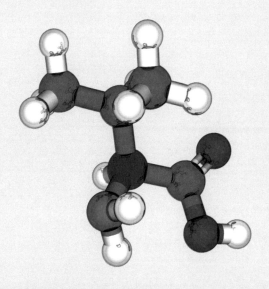

Type	Properties		Sources
branched non polar hydrophobic	MW - 117.15	essential glucogenic	**animal:** most meats & protein foods **plant:** soy beans
	forms sterols in muscles & AT ↑ muscle grth	in sickle cell anaemia substitutes for the polar glutamate & causes RBCs to agglutinate	related to Isoleucine, Leucine

Calcium regulation

Calcium is essential for: blood clotting, enzyme activation & regulation, muscle contraction including cardiac muscle & N transmissions. It takes up about 2% of body wgt - most of which is stored in the bones & teeth.

Because of Ca's role in N transmission & muscle contraction the B[Ca] must be very tightly controlled, even at the cost of bone strength.

Ca needs Vita C & D for adequate absorption, re-sorption from the kidney & maintenance of serum levels.

extracellular concentrations of Ca	↓ ○	↑ ●
PTH	↑	↓
absorption of Ca from the GIT CA	+++	blocked
release of Ca from the bone CB	+++	blocked
re-absorption of Ca from the kidney with excretion of PO_4^{3-} CR	+++	blocked
Calcitonin	↓	↓

A	**Extracellular fluid**
B	**Thyroid & Parathyroid glands (posterior view)**
CA	**GIT - site of Ca absorption**
CB	**bone - site of Ca storage**
CR	**kidney site of Ca re-sorption / excretion**

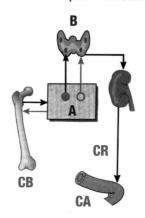

Differential Diagnoses of Hypercalcaemia

Condition	Calcium Blood levels	Calcium Urine levels	Phosphate Blood levels	Alkaline Phosphatase (Indicates bone metabolism)	Other Findings
1° Carcinoma – not bone	◀	◀	▼■	▲	lung cancer bronchogenic
Carcinoma – 2° to bone	◀	◀	■	□	Lucent X-ray lesions
Disuse atrophy Long standing Immobilization	◀	◀	▲■	■▲	DD OP
Hyperparathyroidism	◀	◀	▶	■▲	sub-periosteal resorption
Milk Alkali syndrome	◀	▶	■	■	alkalosis / ulcer Hx / subcutaneous calcification
Multiple myeloma	◀	◀	■	■▲	Bence – Jones proteins in urine / serum globulin levels ◀
Sarcoidosis	◀	◀	▲■	■▲	serum globulin levels ◀
Thyrotoxicosis	◀	◀	■	■▲	weight loss / hyperactivity
Hypervitaminosis – D	◀	◀	▲■	■	Hx of Vitamin D ingestion

Catecholamine pathways

A formation of dopamine, adrenaline & noradrenaline
B catecholamine structures

L-Phenylalanine (p) is converted into L-Tyrosine (t) by the enzyme **Aromatic amino-acid hydroxylase (1)** (AAAH), with tetrahydrobiopterin as a cofactor & oxygen. This step is repeated to form L-DOPA adding the ferrous ion (Fe^{2+}).

L-DOPA is converted into Dopamine by the enzyme **Aromatic amino-acid decarboxylase (2)** (AADC), with pyridoxal phosphate as the cofactor. Dopamine (i) is also used as precursor in the synthesis of adrenaline (iii) & noradrenaline. Dopamine is converted into noradrenaline (ii) by the enzyme **Dopamine Hydroxylase (3)** (DBH), with Vita C as a cofactor, & then to adrenaline by the enzyme **Phenylethanolamine N-methyltransferase (4)** (PNMT).

The catecholamines are synthesized in the adrenal medulla by the chromaffin cells & the postganglionic N fibres in the SymNS. Dopamine also acts as a neurotransmitter and is produced in the Substatia nigra & ventral tegmental area of the Brainstem.

1 **Aromatic amino-acid hydroxylase - rate limiting step in catecholamine production**

2 **Aromatic amino-acid decarboxylase**

3 **Dopamine hydroxylase**

4 **Phenylethanolamine N-methyltransferase**

5 **Catecholamine-O-methyltransferase** **one of the 2 enzymes which deactivate the catecholamines - the other is** monoamine oxidase (MAO) **- not shown**

  p **L-Phenylalanine**
  t - **L-Tyrosine**
  i - **Dopamine**
  ii - **Noradrenaline**
  iii - **Adrenaline**

A

p

t

i

ii

iii

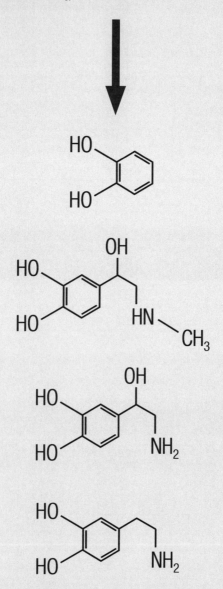

© A. L. Neill

tyrosine

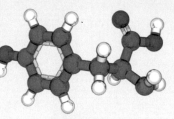

catechol

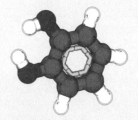

adrenaline

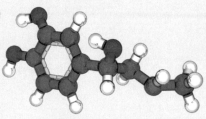

noradrenaline

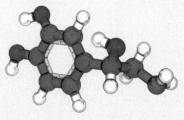

dopamine

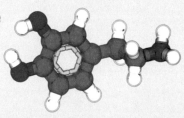

89

Cholesterol Cell Membrane Transport

Esterification of cholesterol

Esterification for transport

Most ingested cholesterol is esterified, which is poorly absorbed, but is a very good form for transport w/n the BS.

Digestive enzymes cleave this ester & the cholesterol passes freely into the enterocytes (intestinal epithelial cells), where it is re-esterified for transport to the liver, via lipoproteins.

Cholesterol is fairly insoluble & confined to the surface of the lipoproteins, but as an ester it can be carried inside the lipoproteins. This vastly ↑ the capacity of lipoproteins, allowing for more efficient cholesterol transport through the BS.

Distinct enzymes catalyze the cholesterol (1) to cholesteryl ester (2) conversion depending on the location of the reaction. **Lecithin:cholesterol acyltransferase (LCAT)** in the PTs, uses phosphatidylcholine (3) as the source of the acyl chain (4)

Acyl-coenzyme A: cholesterol acyltransferase 2 (ACAT2), is found in both the intestine & liver, & uses acyl-CoA (5).

ACAT1 is found in all Ts as a universal transferring enzyme, to abstract small amounts of cholesterol for the cell's use.

Cholesterol is recycled. The liver excretes it in a non-esterified form (via bile) into the GIT.

About 50% of the excreted cholesterol is reabsorbed by the SI into the BS.

1   **cholesterol**
2   **cholesteryl esters**
3   **phosphatidylcholine**
4   **unsaturated FA**
5   **acyl CoA**
6   **acetyl CoA**

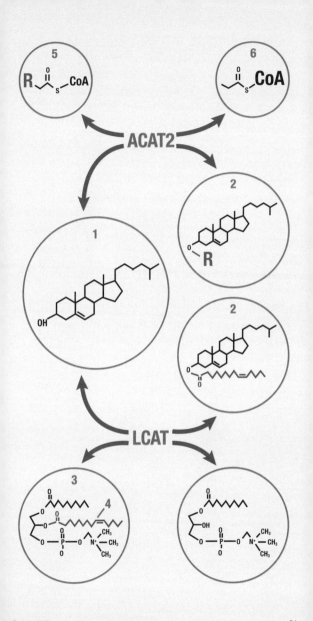

Cholesterol to Steroid Hormones - Overview

A Pregnenolone formation
B DHEA & DHEA-S circulating forms 3D & 2D
C Overview of the pathways to steroid Hs from cholesterol

Enzymes in the Pathways to Steroid Hs -

ACTH activates the pathway from cholesterol to steroid Hs, by permitting transport of cholesterol into the mitochondria through **StAR** - red boxes are placed around internal mitochondrial reactions.

This activates C_{27} **Cholesterol** → C_{21}**-Pregnenolone**. the most important & rate limiting step, of steroid H synthesis controlled by the *primary P450 cytochrome - cholesterol side chain cleavage enzyme* (P450ssc AKA CYP11A1).

Steroids with 21 C atoms = PREGNANES
Steroids with 19 C atoms = ANDROSTANES / TESTOSTERONES
Steroids with 18 C atoms = OESTRANES / OESTROGENS

The most abundant circulating steroid H is DHEA. It is produced primarily in the adrenal cortex, & circulates in balance as an inactive sulphonated storage form (DHEA-S).

DHEA AKA androstenolene is directly active as an androgen but is also a substrate for further modification to more effective sex Hs.

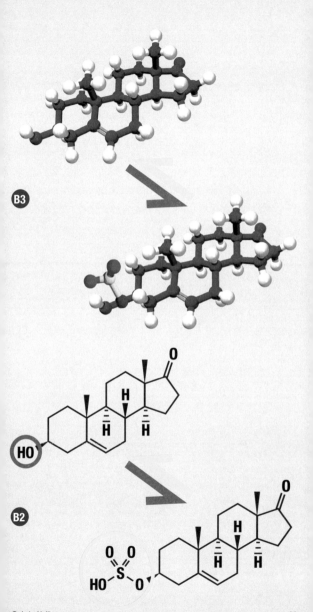

B3

B2

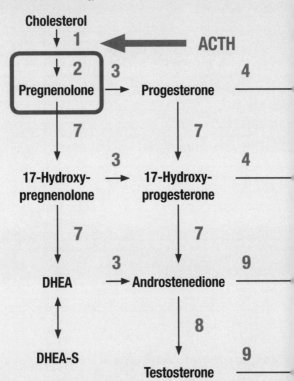

androgens

MINERALOCORTICOCOIDS

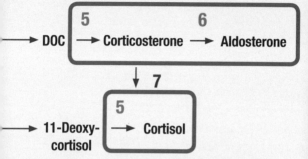

DOC ⟶ Corticosterone ⟶ Aldosterone

11-Deoxy-cortisol ⟶ Cortisol

GLUCOCORTICOCOIDS

oestrogens

Oestrone

SEX HORMONES

8

Oestradiol

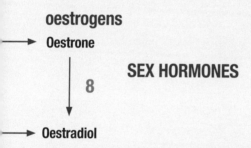

Enzyme Number	Enzyme Name*
1	Steroidgenic acute regulatory protein (StAR)
2	Cholesterol side chain cleavage enzyme
3	3β-Hydroxylase dehydrogenase
4	21α-Hydroxylase
5	11β-Hydroxylase
6	Corticosterone Methyloxidase
7	17α-Hydroxylase
8	17β-Hydroxysteroid dehydrogenase
9	Aromatase

* Please note only one name for an enzyme or substrate is used but
alternatives are listed in detail in the abbreviation section

Cholesterol

Schema of the Adrenal cortex
Schema of the Ovary
Schema of the seminiferous tubules of the Testis

Precursor to Steroid Hs -

Cholesterol is the commonest steroid in the body & the basis of all steroid Hs, which are synthesized in:

the 3 zones of the adrenal cortex, ZG, ZF & ZR   **1**

the ovaries - granulosa cells   **2**

the testes -interstitial cells (AKA Leydig cells)   **3**

ZG synthesises the ALDOSTERONE, the main Mineralocorticoid & the only site of production.

ZF synthesises the CORTISOL & CORTICOSTERONE - the main Glucocorticosteroids also synthesised in the ZR

ZR is the primary site of the ANDROSTENEDIONE the common precursors for the sex Hs, & DHEA the most abundant circulating steroid, - & steroid H substrate.
It also produces limited amounts of TESTOSTERONE

The granulosa **(G)** cells of the ovary produce the OESTROGENS until ovulation

After ovulation the **CL** - produces PROGESTERONE.

The ovary is also the site of TESTOSTERONE synthesis in the female.

The interstitial cells (**cells of Leydig - (L)**) of the testes lying b/n the seminiferous tubules **(S)** produce TESTOSTERONE, & the Sertoli cells **(Se)** produce OESTRADIOL

The steroid Hs are primarily regulated by ACTH produced in the ant. pituitary gland.

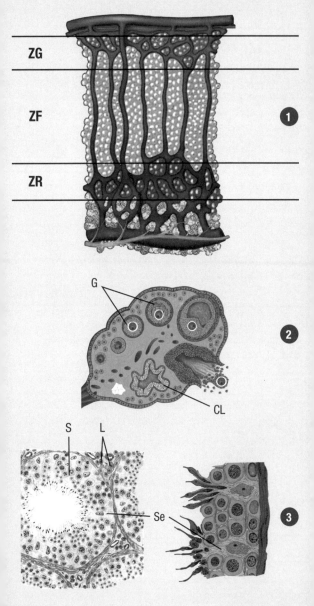

ZG

ZF

ZR

1

G

2

CL

S   L

Se

3

© A. L. Neill

Cholesterol

$C_{27}H_{46}O$ - a modified organic steroid

AKA 2,15-dimethyl-14-(1,5-dimethylhexyl) tetracyclo[8.7.0.0^{2,7}.0^{11,15}]heptadec-7-en-5-ol

3D structural representations
2D chemical formulae
2D structural representations

Structure - A 27 Carbon molecule with:

a polar hydrophilic head (hydroxyl group)	**1**
a middle rigid 4 sterol ring structure (steroid)	**2**
a flexible hydrophobic hydrocarbon tail (lipid)	**3**

This structure allows it to intertwine with the phospholipids of membranes & apolipoproteins, while interacting with the surrounding watery solute i.e. blood or lymph, & its proteins.

This structure is the basis of all steroid Hs, is the main bile salt, and ingredient of Vita D an essential ingredient of all membranes in or around each cell, including ic transport eg endocytosis & has antioxidant properties. It is poorly soluble in water.

Cholesterol is essential for all animal life, & can be synthesised in each cell. Total body-cholesterol is b/n 30-40 g with the total body-cholesterol synthesis ~1g/day.

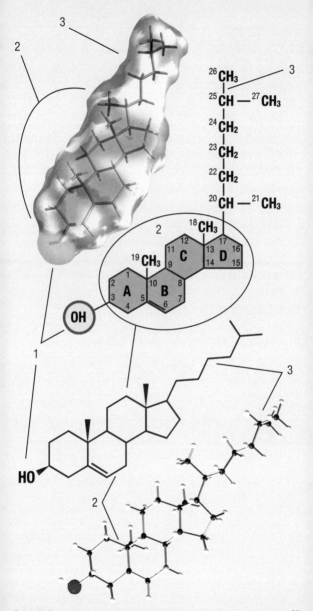

3

2

26 CH₃
25 CH — 27 CH₃
24 CH₂
23 CH₂
22 CH₂
20 CH — 21 CH₃

3

2

18 CH₃
19 CH₃   12
                11   13   17   16
                  C   D   15
                9   8
    1   10   14
  2   A   5   B   6   7
  3   4

OH

1

3

HO

2

© A. L. Neill

Cholesterol

Pathway of synthesis from acetyl CoA

Biosynthesis - Acetyl CoA formed from the oxidation of FAs or pyruvate in the mitochondria, OR from acetate or ethanol in the cytoplasm & it is the precursor of cholesterol.

The rate limiting irreversible step of cholesterol synthesis is when *HMG-CoA-reductase* converts (acetyl CoA) X3 ➜ 3 hydroxy-3-methylglutaryl-CoA (HMG-CoA). *(*site of action of most statin drugs)*

The process of cholesterol synthesis has five major steps:

1. **Acetyl-CoAs X3 are converted to 3-hydroxy-3-methylglutaryl-CoA (HMG-CoA)**

2. **HMG-CoA is converted to mevalonate**

3. **Mevalonate is converted to the isoprene based molecule, isopentenyl pyrophosphate (IPP), losing CO2**

4. **IPP is converted to squalene**

5. **Squalene is converted to cholesterol**

Regulation of cholesterol synthesis

The cellular supply of cholesterol is maintained at a steady level by 3 distinct mechanisms:

1. **Regulation of HMG-CoA activity & levels**

2. **Regulation of excess ic free cholesterol through ACAT**

3. **Regulation of plasma[cholesterol] levels via LDL receptor-mediated uptake & HDL-mediated reverse transport.**

The LDL receptor scavenges circulating LDL from the BS, whereas *HMG-CoA reductase* leads to an ↑ of endogenous production of cholesterol.

Cholesterol synthesis is halted when ATP levels are low, &/or exogenous cholesterol levels are high.

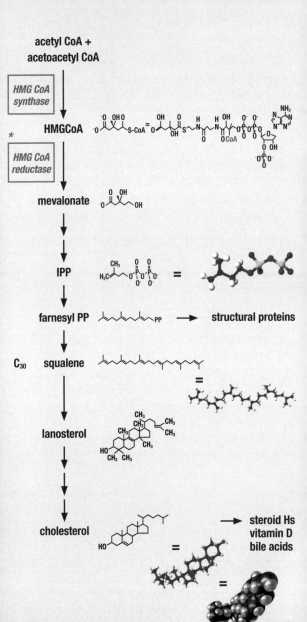

acetyl CoA +
acetoacetyl CoA

HMG CoA synthase

HMGCoA

*

HMG CoA reductase

mevalonate

IPP

farnesyl PP → structural proteins

C$_{30}$ squalene

lanosterol

cholesterol → steroid Hs
vitamin D
bile acids

© A. L. Neill

101

Erythropoietin (EPO)
AKA haematopoietin AKA haemopoietin

Schema EPO regulating erythropoiesis
Non haematopoietic roles of EPO

EPO's major function is to control erythropoiesis, or RBC production. In the presence of hypoxia levels may increase 1000X & signal the RBM to produce more precursors of RBC e.g. pro-erythroblasts, while also protecting RBCs from programmed cell death - apoptosis, in the RBM, liver & spleen.

EPO has other functions. It helps prevent the formation of foam cells from monocytes, by ↓ their ability to take up LDLs, & its anti-IF effects protects damaged neurological & cardiovascular T, particularly in AI diseases.

1 **↓ levels of O2 in the B...**
2 **are detected by the kidneys (JGA & MD cells)**
3 **which stimulate renal peritubular & glomerular mesangial cells to produce EPO**
4 **↑ circulating EPO ...**
5 **activates RBM to ...**
6 **↑ RBC production, ↑ O₂ carrying capacity in the B**
7 **EPO also ↑ rate of wound healing due to its**
8 **stimulation of angiogenesis, which protects**
9 **cardiovascular T**
10 **neural T including the Brain &**
11 **the retina**

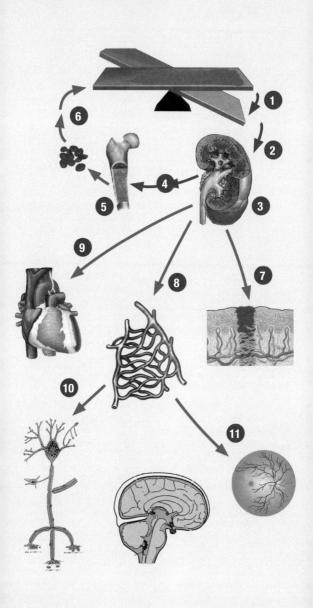

Erythropoietin (EPO) 2
AKA haematopoietin AKA haemopoietin

A   Structure of EPO - glycosylated
B   Major sites of synthesis of EPO - Kidney
C   Supplementary site of EPO synthesis - Liver

EPO is at least 40% glycosylated in circulation with the number and types of sugars ie its various glyoforms modulating its effects. It is produced by the interstitial fibroblasts in the kidney, mesangial cells (7) in close association with peritubular capillaries & tubular epithelium (4), & it has quite diverse effects on different Ts, possibly because of these different forms. It is also produced in peri-sinusoidal cells of the liver.

1   **high mannose oligosaccharide, bonded to the EPO in this glycoform, via N bonds**
2   **single glycan - O-linked**
3   **JGA / c = periarteriolar cells of the JGA**
4   **tubular cells / d = DCT / p = PCT / c = collecting ducts**
5   **arterioles / a = afferent / e = efferent / c = peritubular capillaries**
6   **MD**
7   **mesangial cells**
8   **perisinusoidal cells AKA stellate cells AKA Ito cells**
9   **endothelial cells + space of Disse**
10 **central vein**
11 **hepatocyte**
12 **Kupfer cell**
13 **hepatic arteriole**
14 **portal vein**
15 **bile duct**

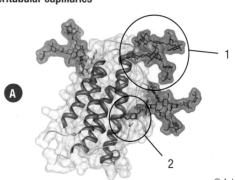

© A. L. Neill

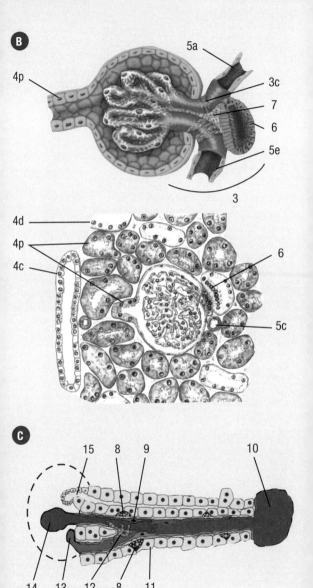

Fatty Acids (FAs) & Triglycerides (TGs)

representations of FAs

FAs are carboxylic acids with a long aliphatic chain (straight hydrocarbon chain). If the bonds b/n the C & H are all single then the FA is *saturated* & each C in the chain has 4 covalent bonds. If there are any 2X bonds b/n the C atoms then the FA is *unsaturated* & has the potential to covalently bind to further atoms.

With the *unsaturated* FAs they may be a "straight" line & hence they are *trans* FAs or "curved" then *cis* FAs. Trans FAs rarely occur in natural oils or fats.

The type of FA is determined by the site of the first unsaturated bond. Counting from the methyl end - if it is on the 3rd C atom then it is an omega 3 FA.

Polyunsaturated bonds cause curving of the molecule.

Free Fatty Acids (FFAs) are those FAs which are not bound to glycerol or other carrier substance. Most FAs are bound to glycerol in the body forming TGs.

1 **saturated FA showing C-H individual bonds**
2 **carboxyl group representations**
3 **unsaturated bond - causing bend - i.e. unsaturated cis FA**
4 **Palmitic FA**
5 **Oleic FA - monounsaturated FA**
6 **Linolenic FA**
7 **Arachidonic FA**
    c = curved representation
    s = 3D representation

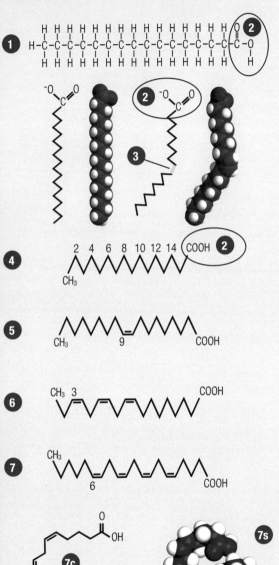

Fatty Acids (FAs) & Triglycerides (TGs)

A representations of TGs

B analysis of the TG structure and component FAs

Triglycerides (TGs) AKA Triacylglycerols, or Triacylglycerides
are made when glycerol & 3 FAs combine forming ester bonds &
liberating water.

The TGs **(1)** have a glycerol back bone **(2)** & 3 FA arms **(3)** which
vary with the person's diet.   In this case palmitic acid **(3i)** a fully
saturated FA more common in plant fats; oleic acid **(3ii)** with a single
2X bond **(4)** & α-linolenic acid **(3iii)** a poly unsaturated FA, commoner
in animal fats. The arms of the TG may "swing around" changing
shape & allow the molecule to take many shapes particularly with the
longer FA chains.

The 3 hydroxy (-OH) grps **(5)** form ester bonds **(6)** with the carboxyl
grps (-COOH) **(7)** of the FAs cleaving off the hydrogen & oxygen
radicals which combine to form 1 water molecule for each bond **(8)**.
Because of their structure TGs can circulate freely in the B moving
through most cm w/o specific transport systems, allowing for the
bidirectional flow of fat & glucose b/n the liver & B.

1 **glycerol backbone**
2 **3 FA arms**
3 **FAs**
      i = Palmitic acid
      ii = Oleic acid
      iii = Linolenic acid
4 **unsaturated C to C bond**
5 **hydroxyl grps**
6 **ester bonds**
7 **carboxyl grps**
8 **water = H_2O**

$C_{55}H_{98}O_6$

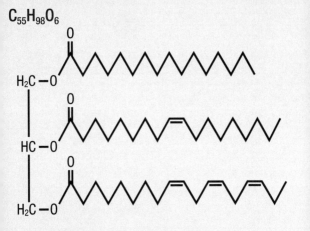

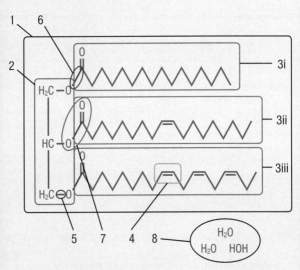

$HOCH_2CH(OH)CH_2OH$ (glycerol) + $R'CO_2H$
(FAi) + $R''CO_2H$ (FAii) + $R'''O_2H$ (FAiii) →
$RCO_2CH_2CH(O_2CR')CH_2CO_2R''$ (TG) + $3H_2O$

HORMONE LIST A to Z

Adipose T (AT) - adipocytes

Adrenal cortex - ZF, ZG, ZR

Corpus luteum (CL)

Ovary - granulosa cells

Placenta - trophoblasts

Prostate gland

Sex Organs

Testes – Leydig cells, sertoli cells

Uterus - decidua, myometrium

Bones - osteoblasts, osteoclasts

Parathyroid Gland (PT) - parafollicular cells, chief cells

Adrenal medulla

Brain - cerebral cortex (CC)

Central nervous system (CNS)

Hypothalamus / neurosecretory Ns / Inhibitory Ns

Pineal gland

Ant. Pituitary gland (Ant. Pit.) - gonadotrophs, lactotrophs, melanotrophs, pars intermedia somatotrophs

Duodenum (Duo)

Gastrointestinal tract (GIT) - mucosa

Small intestine (SI) - K cells

Stomach

Endothelium - vascular

Hair follicle (HF)

Platelets

Skin

Thymus

White blood cells (WBCs)

Heart - atrial cells, cardiomyocytes

Kidney (Ky)

DCT, JGA, macula densa, PCT

Pancreas

Salivary gland

Liver - perisinusoidal cells

Post. Pituitary (Post. Pit.) neurosecretary Ns

Skeletal muscle (SKM)

Smooth Muscle (SM)

Thyroid gld - thyrotrophs, parafollicular cells, C cells

NOTES ON THIS TABLE

1 The terms, peptide & H are sometimes used interchangeably, for small Hormones. As far as possible the more familiar term is used with the other listed.

2 **Trophic** (Brit.) **(TROH-fik) & tropic** (US) **(TROH- pik)** both meaning *stimulating the activity of another endocrine gland* are interchangeable suffixes; for clarity only trophic is used here; hence gonadotrophs = gonadotropes = cells causing growth of the gonads.

3 Many Hs act on other Hs before there is a bodily / cellular response, 2° Hs. These are referred to as releasing or inhibiting factors, RFs or IFs wherever possible.

A

Hormone (Abbreviation)	Structure CLASS/TYPE	Principal Source	Main effects (Target Ts)
5-hydroxytryptamine AKA Serotonin (5HT)			
ADIPOKINES **ADIPOCYTOKINES**	group of AT derived Hs	AT - fat cells	see indiv. members of this grp pro-IF Hs
Adiponectin AKA Adipocyte complement factor 1q (ACRP) AKA AdipoQ	protein (117 AAs) 244 AAs with 4 functional domains	AT - fat cells	↓ IR ↑ FFA oxidation
Adrenalin **AKA Adrenaline** **AKA Epinephrine** *see also noradrenalin*	Tyrosine derivative CATECHOLAMINE	Adrenal medulla	classic "fight-or-flight" response, ↑ glycogenolysis, lipid mobilization ↑ SM contraction ↑ HR, ↑ cardiac function binds to all catecholamine receptors (α- & β- adrenergic); throughout the body
Adrenocorticotrophic H (ACTH) **AKA Corticotrophin**	PP (39 AAs) melanocortin	Ant. Pituitary	↑ synthesis of corticosteroids (Adrenal cortex - adrenocortical cells)
Aldosterone	mineraloocorticoid steroids	Adrenal cortex / ZG	↑ B volume, ↑ BP ↑ Na⁺ absorption & ↑ K⁺ & H⁺ secretion (Ky)
Amylin AKA islet amyloid polypeptide (IAPP)	PP (37 AAs)	Pancreas β cells	↓ gastric emptying, ↓ digestive secretion, ↓ food intake ↓ GCG released with INS compliments its actions
Amphiregulin	PP (78 AAs)	Pancreas	competes with EGF

	group of steroid derived Hs	Adrenal cortex Ovaries, Testes	see indiv members of this grp involved in maintenance of sex organs & characteristics
Androgens (e.g., testosterone)	androgen steroids	Adrenal cortex Sex organs	see indiv members of this grp involved in maintenance of sex organs & characteristics
Androstenedione			Substrate for Oestrogen
Angiotensinogen pro-H/inactive	protein (485 AAs)	Liver	present in the α_2-globulin fraction of plasma cleaved by **Renin** to form Angiotensin I
Angiotensinogen -I pro-H/partially active	PP (10 AAs)	Kidney	the C-terminal 2 AAs are cleaved by **Angiotensin-Converting Enzyme, ACE** to form Angiotensin II
Angiotensinogen -II pre H **Angiotensin (AGT)**	PP (8 AAs)	Kidney	↑ vasoconstriction, ↑ BP essential hypertension ↑ release of Aldosterone
Anti-diuretic H AKA Vasopressin (ADH)	PP (9 AAs)	Hypothalamus synthesizes the H Post. Pit. releases the H	↑ cardiomyocyte contractility (Heart) ↑ glycogenolysis (Liver) ↑ water reabsorption (renal DCT) ↑ vasodilation / ↓ BP (arterioles) ↑ ACTH (Ant Pit.)
Anti-Müllerian H AKA Müllerian inhibiting H (AMH) AKA Anti-Paramesonephric H	glycoprotein TRANSFORMING GFs	Ovaries / granulosa cells Testes / Sertoli cells	↓ TRH, ↓ prolactin suppresses formation of Müllerian ducts in ♂ embryo / maintains follicles throughout ♀ reproductive life
Atrial Naturetic H (ANP) AKA atrial naturetic peptide	**pre-H** 126 AAs PP (28, 32)	Heart - cardiomyocytes	↓ BP by: ↓ SM / ↓ PVR (arteries) ↓ Aldosterone

B

Hormone (Abbreviation)	Structure CLASS/TYPE	Principal Source	Main effects (Target Ts)
Betatrophin AKA β tropin	protein (193 AAs)	Liver	
Bone γ-carboxyglutamic acid-containing protein (BGLAP) AKA Osteocalcin			
Brain Naturetic H AKA Brain Naturetic peptide (BNP)	PP	Brain	↓ BP by: ↓ PVR (less effective than ANP)

C

Hormone (Abbreviation)	Structure CLASS/TYPE	Principal Source	Main effects (Target Ts)
Calciferol AKA Vita D2 *see also Vita D*	steroid derivative (secosteroid - sterol)	**Sunshine**; Skin, Liver & Ky combined for synthesis	Ca & PO₄ homeostasis less effective than Calcitriol
Calcitonin (CT)	PP (32 AAs)	Thyroid Gland parafollicular C cells	↑ bone synthesis ↓ B[Ca] phosphate regulation tied to Ca
Calcitonin gene-related peptide (CGRP)	PP (37 AAs)	Thyroid Gland parafollicular C cells *alternative product to Calcitonin*	vasodilator not as active as Calcitonin
Calcitriol (Vita D3) active *Calcidiol - inactive form (Vita D3)*	C9-10 secosteroid derived from Cholesterol	**Sunshine**, Skin, Liver & Ky-PCT combined for synthesis	↑ Vita D₃ - active form ↑ absorption Ca / PO₄ (GIT & Ky) ↓ PTH ↑ bone mineralization

© A. L. Neill

CATECHOLAMINES	group of Tyrosine derived Hs	Adrenal Medulla	see indiv. members of this grp involved in Fight or Flight in conjunction with the SymNS
Cholecystokinin (CCK)	PPs (8 - 33 AAs)	Duodenum Stomach	↑ digestive enzymes (Pancreas - exocrine cells) ↑ bile flow (GB contractions) ↑ hunger (cerebral hunger centre)
Chorionic gonadotropin (HCG)		Placenta - syncytiotrophoblasts	similar to LH
Chorionic somatomammotropin AKA Placental lactogen (hPL)	protein (191 AAs)	Placenta - trophoblasts	similar to : Prolactin, GH only present in preg. peaks at term ↑ maternal BMRt
Chromogranin A AKA Parathyroid secretory H	protein (439 AAs)	Adrenal medulla Pancreas / β cells	↑ synthesis of secretory vesicles in their own & nearby cells precursors of the agents which promote their release - functional peptides
Corticotropin AKA Adrenocorticotropin H (ACTH)			
Corticotropin-releasing factor (CRF)	PP (41 AAs)	Hypothalamus	↑ ACTH / (Ant. Pituitary) ↑ lipotropin → ↑ endorphins (CC)
Cortisol	glucocorticoid steroids	Adrenal cortex - ZF / ZR	↑ gluconeogenesis ↑ glucose uptake (SKM & WAT) ↑ B [AA] / ↑ FFAs - i.e. lipolysis (WAT) IFR & IMR anti-inflammatory
Cortistatin (CORT) *similar to somatostatin (SIF)*	neuropeptide PP (105 AAs) similar to SRIF	CC - inhibitory Ns	↓ N activity; ↑ slow-wave sleep; (CC amygdala, hippocampus) ↓ locomotor activity

D

Hormone (Abbreviation)	Structure CLASS/TYPE	Principal Source	Main effects (Target Ts)
Dehydroepiandersterone (DHEA) AKA Didehydroepiandrosterone Androstenolone AKA Prasterone (INN)	androgen steroids / neurosteroid *most abundant steroid in the BS*	Adrenal cortex Brain Ovary / theca cells Testes / Leydig cells	↑ virilization ↑ anabolic grth
Dihydrotestosterone (DHT) AKA 5-DHT AKA Androstanolone 5-α-dihydrotestosterone 1° androgen in the adult	androgen steroids *(metabolite of Testosterone)* *(in the ♂ it cannot be converted to oestradiol so remains higher longer- hence male pattern baldness)*	Adrenal cortex Hair follicles (HFs) Prostate Testes	↑ cell grth / maturation ↑ cell mitosis (bulbourethral gld, penis, prostate gld, scrotum, seminal vesicles) Testosterone → 5-DHT w/in the target cell bc it needs high conc. to work high levels cause male pattern baldness ↑ prostate size/ low levels maintain HFs Essential role in formation of ♂ embryo 's external genitals, & maintenance in the adult
Dopamine AKA Prolactin inhibiting factor (PIF)	CATECHOLAMINE neurotransmitter as well as H	Adrenal Medulla Brain Hypothalamus	↑ movement, SKM contractility ↓ lactation involved in pleasure & reward - drugs of abuse either

E

Hormone (Abbreviation)	Structure CLASS/TYPE	Principal Source	Main effects (Target Ts)
Enkephalin	protein	Brain	regulate pain
Endorphins	PP - from lipotropins	Ant. Pit.	↑ mood
Endothelin	PP (21 AAs)	Endothelium - vascular	↑ contraction of medium sized BVs ↑ contractions in the stomach (SM)
Enteroglucagon AKA Glucagon-like peptide (GLP-1)			
Enterostatin	derived from pancreatic colipase (PP 5 AAs)	AT / Fat cells GIT	→ high fat diet (but not a low fat diet)
Epinephrine AKA Adrenaline			
Epithelial growth factor (EGF)	PP (55 AAs)	Salivary glands	↑ epithelial lining repairs (GIT, skin) regulated by inorganic iodine ↓ gastric & protease secretions
Erythropoietin (EPO) AKA Haemopoietin AKA Haematopoietin	glycoprotein (166 AAs)	Bones Ky - peritubular cells Liver / peri-sinusoidal cells	↑ RBC production (RBM) ↑ wound healing (skin), neuroprotection from hypoxia (Brain)
Estrogen AKA Oestrogen			

F

Hormone (Abbreviation)	Structure CLASS/TYPE	Principal Source	Main effects (Target Ts)
Fibroblast Growth Factors 23 (FGF-23) AKA Phosphatonin	protein (251)	Bone	↑ synthesis of CT
Fibroblast Growth Factors 23 (FGF-23) AKA Phosphatonin	protein (216)	Ileum	synthesis of bile acids ↑ filling of the GB (relaxes the SM) ↑ glycogen formation
Follicle-stimulating H (FSH)	protein (204) α-FSH 96 AAs β-FSH 120 AAs	Ant. Pit.	♀: ↑ maturation of Graäfian follicles (Ovary). ↑ oestrogen ♂: ↑ spermatogenesis ↑ production of androgen binding protein (Testes - Sertoli cells)

G

Hormone (Abbreviation)	Structure CLASS/TYPE	Principal Source	Main effects (Target Ts)
Galanin (GAL)	neuropeptide (29 AAs)	CNS GIT	modulation & ↓ AP in Ns neuromodulator
Gastric inhibitory polypeptide (GIP) AKA Glucose-dependent-insulinotropic PP (GIP)			
Gastrin	PP (17-34 AAs)	Stomach	↑ gastric acid, pepsin (Stomach - parietal cells AKA acid producing cells) ↑ pancreatic enzymes

© A. L. Neill

117

Gastrin-releasing peptide (GRP)	neuropeptide PP (27 AAs)	postganglionic Ns of the Vagus N	↑ gastrin (stomach - G cells) ↑ CCK (SI neuroenteroendocrine I cells)
Ghrelin antagonists **Leptin Obestatin**	PP (28 AAs)	GIT	↑ appetite, ↑ secretion of GH (Ant. Pit.) ↑ INS (Pancreas β cells) ↑ gastric emptying ↑ glomerulotopin
GLUCOCORTICOIDS (e.g. cortisol corticosterone)	steroids	Adrenal cortex	**see individual members of this grp** → IFR, IMR → protein synthesis
Glucagon (GCG) antagonist **INS**	PP (29 AAs)	Pancreas / α cells	↑ glycogenolysis & ↑ gluconeogenesis (Liver) ↑ lipolysis, ↑ B [glucose] → INS
Glucagon-like peptide (GLP-1) AKA Enteroglucagon	PP (30 & 31 AAs)	GIT	↑ INS, ↓ GCG, ↓ gastric emptying
Glucose-dependent-insulinotrophic PP (GIP) AKA Gastric Inhibitory PP	PP (42 AAs)	Intestine / K cells	→ gastric acid (stomach / G cells) ↑ INS (Pancreas / β cells)
Gonadotropin-releasing H (GnRH) AKA Luteinizing H releasing factor (LHRF)	PP (10 AAs)	Hypothalamus	↑ FSH, ↑ LH (Ant. Pit. / gonadotrophs)

Hormone (Abbreviation)	Structure CLASS/TYPE	Principal Source	Main effects (Target Ts)
Growth H (GH) AKA Somatotrophin	protein (191 AAs)	Ant. Pit.- somatotrophs	↑ growth/anabolic ↑ cell mitosis (all cells in the body) ↑ sulphation of bone ↑ IGF-1 (Liver)

H

Hormone (Abbreviation)	Structure CLASS/TYPE	Principal Source	Main effects (Target Ts)
Haemopoietin AKA Erythropoietin			
Hepcidin antagonist EPO	PP (25 AAs)	Liver	↓ iron export from cells (all cells in the body)
Histamine		Stomach	vasoconstriction (BVs) ↑ contractions of SM (Stomach)
Human chorionic gonadotropin (hCG) placenta equiv of LH similar to TSH	protein (237 AAs)	Placenta - Trophoblast	↑ maintenance of CL in early pregnancy ↓ IMR, towards the human embryo (immune Ts - LNs) ↑ TH (thyroid)
Human placental lactogen HPL	protein	Placenta	↑ INS & IGF-1 ↑ IR & ↑ CHO intolerance

I

Hormone (Abbreviation)	Structure CLASS/TYPE	Principal Source	Main effects (Target Ts)
Incretins	PPs (31, 42)	Duodenum Stomach	potentiating effects of INS (all cells in the body) ↓ GCG (pancreas)
Inhibin A & B	A protein (134 AAs) B protein (115 AAs) TRANSFORMING GFs	Ovary / granulosa cells Placenta / foetal trophoblasts Testes / Sertoli cells	↓ FSH (Ant. Pit.)
Insulin (INS) antagonist GCG	PP - 2 subunits 2α + 2β (51 AAs = 21 + 30 PPs bonded)	Pancreas / β cells	↑ cellular uptake glucose, & lipids cells from the B (SKM) ↑ glycogeneogenesis (Liver) ↑ glycolysis (Liver & SKM) ↑ lipids ↑ synthesis TGs from adipocytes ↑ anabolic processes (all cells)
Insulin-like growth factors-1 &2 (IGF-1) AKA Somatomedin	PP (70 AAs)	Liver / hepatocytes	same effects as INS, but much less potent regulate cell growth & development (all cells/organs)
Irisin	protein (112 AAs)	SKM (induced by PGs)	conversion WAT → BAT
Islet amyloid polypeptide (IAPP) AKA Amylin			

J

K

L

Hormone (Abbreviation)	Structure CLASS/TYPE	Principal Source	Main effects (Target Ts)
Leptin (LEP) antagonist - Grehlin	protein (167 AAs) precursor to the active 146 AAs	Liver Fat cells (adipocytes) Hypothalamus GIT Placenta	↓ appetite (cerebral T) ↑ metabolism (all cells) ↑ IFR ↑ BP ↑ bone mass *may initiate puberty*
Leukotrienes	eicosanoids	WBCs	↑ vascular permeability (Endothelium - vascular)
LIPOTROPINS (LPH) eg β lipotropin	PPs β-PPs = 93AAs γ-PPs = 60 AAs	Ant. Pituitary - fragments of the long PP which also forms ACTH	↑ lipolysis ↑ FAs (AT) ↑ steroidogenesis, (adrenal cortex) ↑ melanin (melanocytes)
Luteinizing H (LH) *similar to hCG TSH*	protein (204 AAs) α-LH 96 AAs β-LH 120 AAs	Ant. Pit. - gonadotrophs	♀: ↑ ovulation / ↑ progesterone (Ovary - follicles) ♂: ↑ testosterone / (Testes - Leydig cells) ↑ interstitial cell dev *may initiate puberty*
Luteinizing H releasing factor (LHRF) AKA Gonadotropin releasing factor			

M

Hormone (Abbreviation)	Structure CLASS/TYPE	Principal Source	Main effects (Target Ts)
Melanin-concentrating H (MCH)	PP (19 AAs)	Hypothalamus	↑ appetite

© A. L. Neill

121

Hormone (Abbreviation)	Structure CLASS/TYPE	Principal Source	Main effects (Target Ts)
Melanocyte Stimulating H (MSH)	PPs melanocortin (α- MSH = 12 PPs strongest β- MSH = 13 γ-MSH = 18)	Ant. Pit.	↓ appetite (Hypothalamus) ↓ IFR, IMR, ↓ cytokines & their receptors (m0, monocytes dendritic cells), darkening of pigment (hair & skin)
Melatonin (MT)	tryptophan derivative (AA)	Pineal gland Ovary	↑↓ circadian rhythm (CNS Peripheral Ts) ↓ oxidative stress → ROS ↑ germ cell & placental protection
MINERALOCORTICOIDS (e.g. Aldosterone)	steroids	Adrenal cortex	maintenance of salt & H_2O balance
Motilin (MLN)	PP (22 AAs)	SI	↑ gastric activity peristalsis (Stomach) ↑ GB contractions (SM)
Müllerian inhibiting H AKA Anti-müllerian H			

N

Hormone (Abbreviation)	Structure CLASS/TYPE	Principal Source	Main effects (Target Ts)
Neuromedin B	PP (10 AAs)	Adrenal medulla GIT Pancreas Hypothalamus Ns	↑ gastrin CCK, GIP, INS, ↑ SM contractions ↑ food intake
Neuropeptide Y (NPY) similar to PYY	PPs (36- AAs 5 Y receptors)		↑ appetite during starvation (Hypothalamus) ↑ fat storage → pain / anxiety

Noradrenaline AKA Norepinephrine	CATECHOLAMINE	classic "fight-or-flight" response, ↑ glycogenolysis, lipid mobilization, ↑ SM contraction ↑ HR, cardiac function (heart) binds to all catecholamine receptors (α- & β-adrenergic)

O

Hormone (Abbreviation)	Structure CLASS/TYPE	Principal Source	Main effects (Target Ts)
Obestatin antagonist Grehlin	PP (23 AAs)	GIT	antagonistic to Ghrelin ↓ appetite
Oestrogens e.g. Oestradiol	containing 18 Carbons	Adrenal cortex Ovarian follicle Placenta	maintain ♀ 2° sex charac. maintain the pregnancy ↑ TBH
Oestradiol (E₂)	primary oestrogen steroid	♀: Ovary - granulosa cells ♂: Testes - Sertoli & Leydig cells from the aromatization of testosterone	♀ = formation of 2° sex charac. ↑ endometrial & uterine grth ± breast glandular grth ↑ pheomelanin synthesis ↑ GH, salt & water retention ↑ bone formation ↑ hepatic binding prot. & clotting factors ↑ platelet adhesiveness ↑ HDL, TGs in the B ↑ cholesterol in the bile

Oestriol (E₃)	oestrogen steroid	**Placenta / trophoblasts**	↑ MRt ↔ SKM mass, fat deposition ↔ bone resorption ↔ GIT motility ↔ apoptosis of germ cells
Oestrone	oestrogen steroid	**Ovary / granulosa cells** fat cells	similar actions to the other oestrogens but to a lesser effect
Orexins	neuropeptide single pre-H orexin A 33 AAs orexin B - 28 AAs	Hypothalamus	↑ wakefulness / (↓ REM sleep) ↑ E expenditure, ↑ appetite
Osteocalcin AKA Bone γ-carboxyglutamic acid-containing protein (BGLAP)	protein	**Bone - Osteoblasts**	↑ INS (Pancreas - β cells) ↑ adiponectin (AT) ↑ testosterone (Leydig cells) bone building
Oxyntomodulin	PP (37 AAs) - 1st 29 similar to GCG	**Colon / Stomach / oxyntic cells**	↓ gastric acid secretion similar to GLP-1 & GLP-2 action; ↑ satiety, E consumption ↓ wgt gain competes with GCG receptors & has sim but weaker reactions

| Oxytocin (OXT) | PP (9 AAs) similar to ADH | Post. Pit. magnocellular neurosecretory cells (responds to suckling reflex & oestradiol) | ↑ release breast milk ↑ contraction (Cervix, Uterus & Vagina - SM in orgasm) ↑ trust b/n people. (CC) ↓ steroid synthesis in testes anti-anxiolytic effects (CC) |

P

Hormone (Abbreviation)	Structure CLASS/TYPE	Principal Source	Main effects (Target Ts)
Pancreatic polypeptide (PaP)	PP (36 AAs)	Pancreas - γ cells AKA PP cells	↓ INS (from glucose) ↓ pancreatic enzymes (pancreas endo & exo) ↓ pepsin / gastrin /acid (GIT) ↑ glycogenolysis (Liver) regulates GI motility
Parathyroid hormone (PTH) antagonist Calcitonin (not as strong) *see indiv H listing*	PP (84 AAs)	Parathyroid gld - chief cells	↑ B[Ca] (bone), ↑ osteoclasts numbers & activity (bone) ↑ Ca²⁺ reabsorption (Kidney) (Slightly) ↓ B[PO₄] & ↑ urine[PO₄] : activates Vita D
Peptide Tyrosine Tyrosine, (PYY)	PP (36 AAs)	Pancreas	↓ motility, secretions ↑ satiety (Stomach)
Phosphatonin	protein	Bone / Osteoblasts	↓ B[PO₄]

	Type	Source	Actions / Effects
Pituitary adenylate cyclase-activating peptide (PACAP)	protein	multiple	↑ enterochromaffin-like cells
Placental lactogen AKA Chorionic somatomammotropin			
Progesterone	progesterone / steroid	Adrenal cortex Placenta + CL when pregnant	↑ Endometrial glds ↑ foetal adrenal development ↑ EGF ↑ body core temp. ↑ MRt / BMR ↑ resp. bronchi ↑ cervical mucus ↑ metabolism of lipids ↑ osteoblasts & -cytes ↑ collagen synthesis ↑ myelin ↑ IMR, IFR → myometrium contractility (Labour) → lactation → GB activity → oestrogen
Progestins	progesterone / steroid		mimic progesterone but weaker
Proinsulin	PP - (large PP chain)	Pancreas / β cells	activities of INS but to a lesser extent
Prolactin releasing factor (PIF)	very similar to TRF	Hypothalamus	Release Prolactin (Ant. Pit. - lactotroph)

Prolactin release inhibiting H (PRH) AKA Dopamine		
Prolactin (PRL) AKA Luteotropic H	protein (198 AAs)	Ant. Pit. / lactotrophs Uterus / decidual cells	↑ milk production (Breasts) ↑ sexual gratification after sexual acts (CC)
Prostacylin (PGI2)	eicosanoid	Endothelium - vascular	↑ vascular permeability (self regulating)
Prostaglandins (PG)	eicosanoid	Testes - seminal vesicles	vasodilation / bronchoconstriction / platelet aggregation
PYY$_{3-36}$ similar to NPY	PP (34 AAs)	Adrenal medulla GIT Pancreas Hypothalamus Ns	activities of INS but to a lesser extent ↑ appetite (hypothalamus) ↑ proteases (pancreas) ↑ bile release (GB)

R

Hormone (Abbreviation)	Structure CLASS/TYPE	Principal Source	Main effects (Target Ts)
Relaxin (RLN)	PP	Uterus / decidual cells CL Placenta	↓ SM contractions (Uterus)
Renin is an enzyme	PPs (54 AAs)	Ky - JGA	activates the renin-angiotensin system by producing angiotensin 1 from angiotensinogen
Resistin	pre-protein (108 AAs)	AT / Fat cells	↑ IR ↑ LDL pro-IF assoc. with obesity, DM2 & CV disease
Retinol Binding Protein 4 (RBP4)	protein (~180 AAs)	AT / Fat cells	↑ IR a specific carrier of Vita A in the BS

S

Hormone (Abbreviation)	Structure CLASS/TYPE	Principal Source	Main effects (Target Ts)
Secretin (SCT) *first H to be identified*	PP (27 AAs)	Duodenum / S cells	Secretion of HCO_3 & water - when pH <4.5 (Duodenum / Brünner's glds, Liver, Pancreas exocrine glds) ↑ CCK ↓ gastric juice acid (Stomach)
Serotonin (5HT) AKA 5-hydroxytryptamine AKA Enteramine AKA Thrombocytin	tryptophan derivative	Brain (20%) GIT (80%) / enterochromaffin cells	↓ appetite ↑ motility ↑ vomiting, diarrhoea (GIT) ↑ memory (Brain) ↑ libido ↑ vasoconstrictor (from platelets) ↑ muscle bone fibre grth / (Heart muscle)
SEX HORMONES ANDROGENS OESTOGENS PROGESTERONES	steroid Hs derived from Cholesterol	ADRENAL CORTEX SEX ORGANS	growth & maintenance of gonads sex organs & 2^0 sex Hs
Somatomedin AKA Insulin-like GH			
Somatostatin AKA Somatotropin release, inhibiting factor (SIF) AKA Growth H inhibiting factor (GIF)	PP (14, 28 AAs)	GIT Hypothalamus / neuroendocrine cells Pancreas / δ cells	↓ GH & TRH (Ant. Pit.) ↓ CCK, Gastrin, GIP, Motilin, VIP, enteroglucagon (GIT) ↓ gastric emptying ↓ SM contractions, ↓ BF (GIT) ↓ GCG ↓ INS exocrine secretions (Pancreas)

Somatotrophin AKA GH			
Substance P (SP)	neuropeptide (11 AAs)	CNS GIT	CNS functions ↑ pain (nociception), ↑ salivary prior to vomiting ↑ vasodilatation ↓ bronchoconstriction

T

Hormone (Abbreviation)	Structure CLASS/TYPE	Principal Source	Main effects (Target Ts)
Testosterone	androgen steroids	Adrenal cortex Ovary / thecal cells Testes / Leydig cells -	↑ libido, ↑ anabolic grth, strength) (bone, mu) ↑ bone density ↑ virilising/muscular maturation (1° & 2° sex organs, & their related cells).
Thrombopoietin (TPO)	protein (332 AAs)	Kidney Liver SKM (+ cardiac mu) / myocytes	↑ platelets (RBM - megakaryocytes)
Thromboxane (TXA2)	eicosanoid	platelets	bronchoconstriction vasoconstriction
THYROID HS mixture of T3&T4	mixture of 2 Hs T3 & T4 look up individual Hs tyrosine derivatives	Thyroid	whole body affected ↑ BMR

© A. L. Neill

T

Hormone (Abbreviation)	Structure CLASS/TYPE	Principal Source	Main effects (Target Ts)
Thyroid-stimulating H (TSH) AKA Thyrotropin	PPs (201 AAs) α-PP = 96AAs β-PP = 112	Ant. Pit./ thyrotrophs	↑T_3, T_4 release & synthesis (Thyroid gld)
Thymosin	protein	Thymus	↑ differentiation WBCs- formation of T cells maintains supports ↑ WBCs
Thyrotrophin-releasing factor (TRF)	PP (3 AAs)	Hypothalamus parvocellular neurosecretory cells	↑ TSH (Thyroid) ↑ PRL (Ant. Pit.)
Thyroxine AKA Thyroxin (T_4)	iodinated di-tyrosine derivative (AA)	Thyroid Gland - thyrotrophs	↑ metabolism ↑ BMR (all cells in the body) responds to TSH ↑ oxidations w/n the cells
Triiodothyronine (T_3)	Tyrosine derivative (AA)	Liver	↑ metabolism much stronger than T_4 (all cells in the body)

U

V

Hormone (Abbreviation)	Structure CLASS/TYPE	Principal Source	Main effects (Target Ts)
Vasoactive intestinal peptide (VIP)	PP (28 AAs)	GIT Pancreas Hypothalamus - SCN	↓ SM. vasodilator (BVs) ↑ H₂O & electrolytes ↑ Gastrin & Pepsin (GIT) potent inotrope / chronotope (heart) neurotransmitter in (ANS) regulation of the circadian cyle & prolactin release (SCN)
Vasopressin AKA Anti-diuretic H			

X
Y
Z

Hormones & Age

Most Hs change with age but there are also changes in the target T sensitivity and the rate of the H synthesis / & breakdown.

ORGAN	CHANGES WITH AGE	EFFECTS
adrenal gland cortex	↓ aldosterone ↓ cortisone release but also ↓ cortisone breakdown ↓ dehydroepiandrosterone	↑ orthostatic hypotension levels unaltered - no obvious effect
adrenal gland medulla	adrenaline noradrenaline	no change
hypothalamus	no change	
ovary	↓ oestrogens > 40yo	menopause
kidney	↓ renin	hypertension
pancreas	insulin minor decrease ↑ insulin resistance	↑ B[glucose] > 50yo
parathyroids	may calcify	↑ PTH may cause OP ↓ Calcitonin
pituitary ant / post	maximum size 40yo ↓ in size > 40yo	↑ FSH ↑ LH ↓ GH ↓ prolactin - ↓ libido
testes	↓ testosterone	↓ erection length / frequency ↓ testes
thyroid	develops lumps & nodules ↓ in synthesis & ↓ breakdown slow decrease in BMR with age	THs various - most levels unchanged ♀ 10X more likely to change > ♂ ↓ > 60 yo

Hormones - changes with Puberty

Hormones change with puberty to bring the individual to full sexual and size maturity. The onset of puberty is earlier for girls than boys by approximately 1-3 years, although there is considerable variation. While fairly straight forward for boys it is more complex for girls.

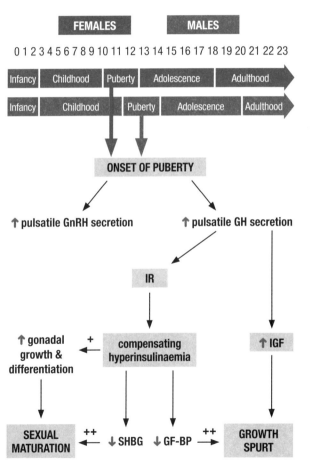

Steroid Hormones I

Main Pathways to steroid Hs in the Adrenal Cortex

The pathway to steroid Hs starts in the mitochondria - indicated by the red squares.

Androstenedione is the common precursor of all the sex Hs.

Most other steps take place in the SER &/or microsomes, requiring transport to & from each area, further moderating the rate of Steroid H synthesis & availability.

CHOLESTEROL

> **cholesterol sidechain cleavage enz**
> **P450ssc**
>
> **1 PREGNENOLONE**

2 PROGESTERONE

3 11-DEOXYCORTICOSTERONE

4 CORTICOSTERONE

> **aldosteron synthase**
> **P450c18**
>
> **5 ALDOSTERONE**

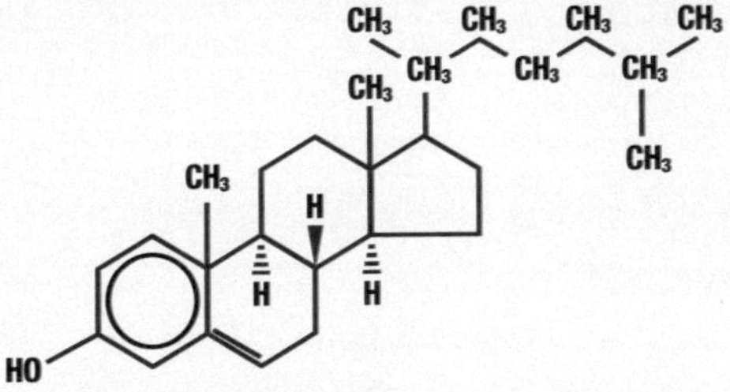

CH3   CH3   CH3   CH3

CH3

CH3

H

H   H

HO

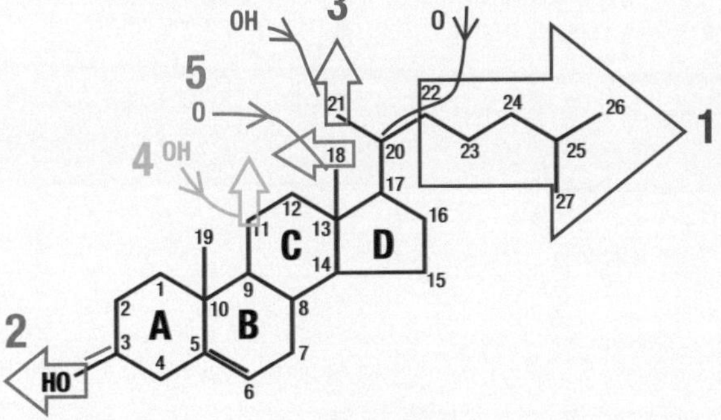

OH   3

5   0   22   0   24   26

O   23   25   1

18   20

21   17

4   OH

11   12   13   16

19   C   D

11   9   14   15

2   1   8

A   10   B   5   7

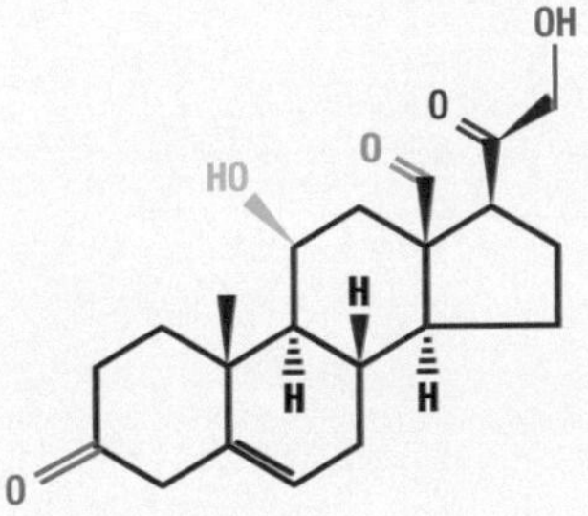

3   6

HO

2

OH

O

HO   O

H

H

O

CHOLESTEROL

cholesterol sidechain cleavage enz
P450ssc

1 PREGNENOLONE

2 17 hydroxyPREGNENOLONE

3 hydroxyPROGESTERONE

4 DHEA ⇌ **4i DHEAS**

P450c17

5 ANDROSTENEDIONE

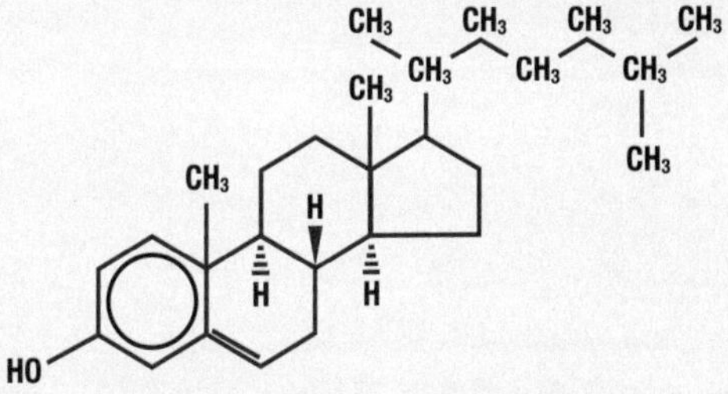

CH₃   CH₃   CH₃   CH₃
   CH₃
CH₃
H
H
HO
H   H

O
4   21
22
24   26
20   23   25
18   27
1
17
12   13   16
11   C   D   OH
19   14   15   2
2   1   9   8
3   A   10   B   5   7
HO   6   O   5
4   5

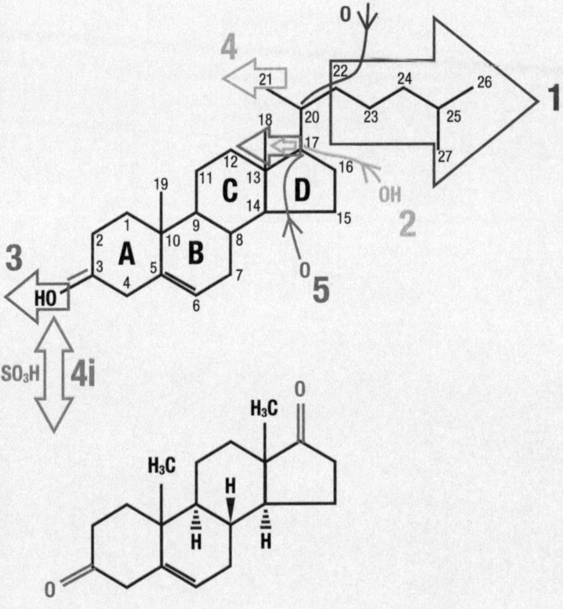

3
HO

SO₃H   4i

H₃C   O

H₃C
H
H   H
O

CHOLESTEROL

cholesterol sidechain cleavage enz
P450ssc

1 PREGNENOLONE

2 PROGESTERONE

3 11-DEOXYCORTICOSTERONE

P450c11

4 CORTICOSTERONE

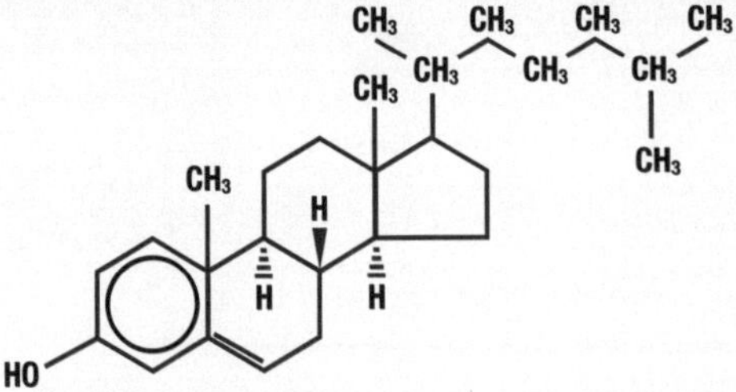

CH₃
CH₃ CH₃ CH₃
CH₃
CH₃
CH₃

H
HO
H H

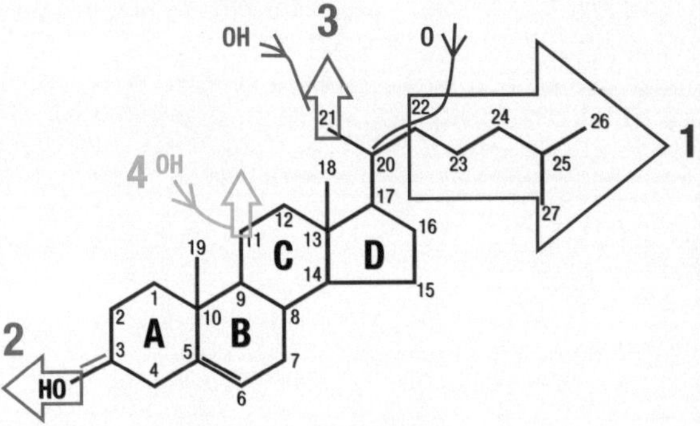

OH 3
O
21 22 24 26
20 23 25 1
18 17
4 OH 16
11 12 13 15
19 C 14 D
2 1 9 8
A 10 B 7
2 3 5 6
HO

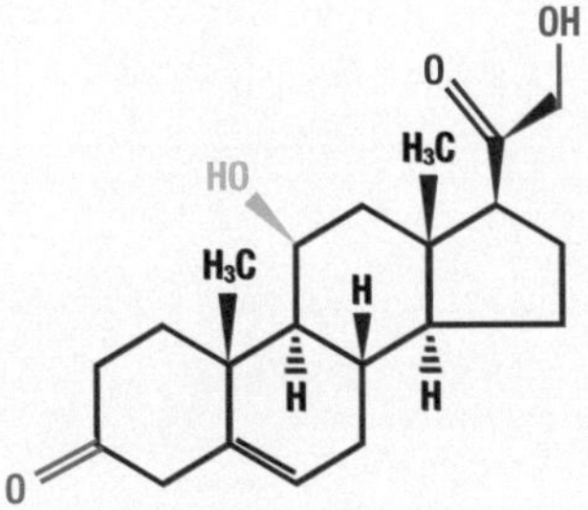

OH
O
H₃C
HO
H₃C
H H
O

CHOLESTEROL

cholesterol sidechain cleavage enz
P450ssc

1 PREGNENOLONE

2 17 hydroxyPREGNENOLONE

3 hydroxyPROGESTERONE

4 11-DEOXYCORTISOL

P450c11

5 CORTISOL

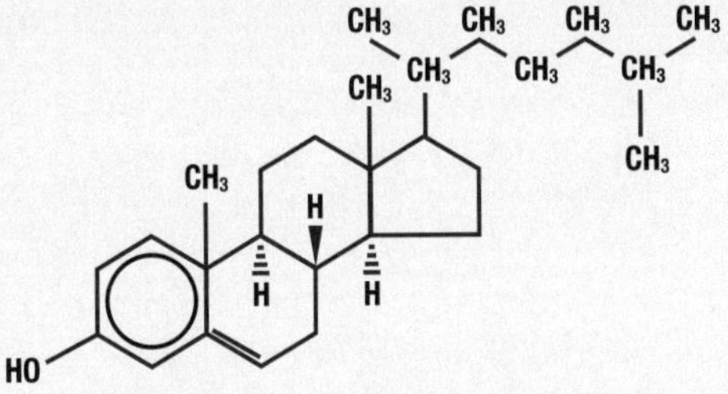

CH₃ CH₃ CH₃ CH₃

CH₃

CH₃

H

H

H

HO

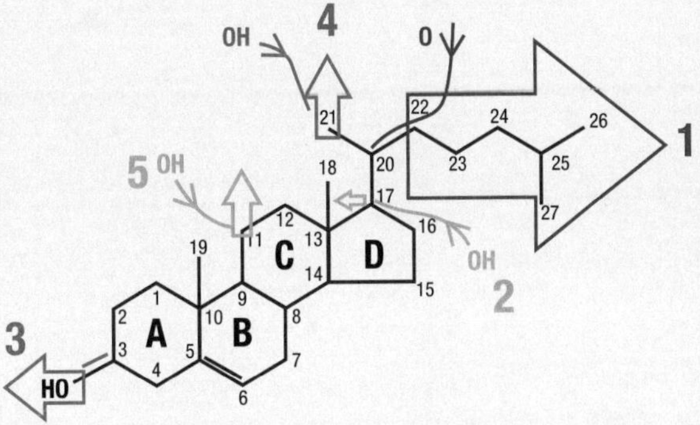

4
OH

1

O

5 OH

18

21

22

24

26

20

23

25

27

2

11

12

13

17

16

OH

C

D

19

10

9

8

14

15

3

2

1

A

B

7

HO

3

4

5

6

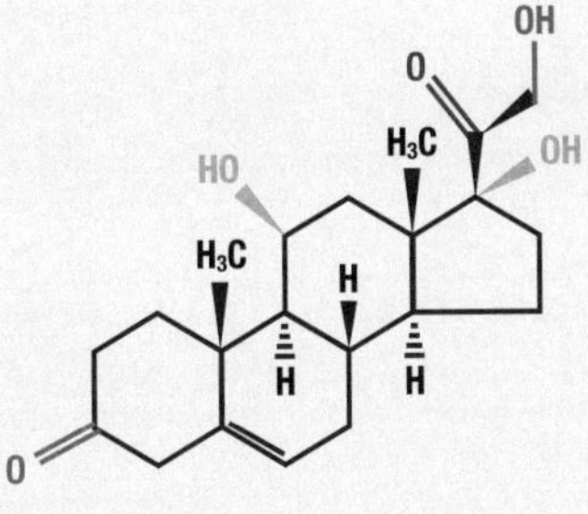

OH

O

H₃C

OH

HO

H₃C

H

H

O

© A. L. Neill

Lipoprotein particles

A   HDL - high density lipoproteins
B   LDL - low density lipoproteins
C   VLDL - very-low density-lipoproteins

Hydrophobic substances need to be transported through the watery B & lymph via special devices.

Lipoprotein particles are the main form of transport of Cholesterol, fats, Steroid Hs & TGAs.

Their composition changes as their contents are taken up by cells & BV walls, & they transform from one form to another.

HDL are the smallest (50-120 Å) & densest (1.06 - 1.2 /gm), containing the most protein & least fat and Cholesterol. These small particles can enter the hepatocytes & are used to form bile salts, which are made up of cholesterol.

LDL - are the major B[cholesterol] carriers. Their surface is covered with apolipoproteins A, C & E which are recognised by the peripheral Ts. These proteins along with cholesterol & fats are ingested leaving the particle lighter & bigger. There are several forms of LDLs.

VLDL - are the largest (> 800 Å) & least dense (< 1.0/gm), containing very little protein. Because of this the cholesterol cannot enter the cells and is ingested by T macrophages which become filled with lipid droplets - FOAM cells.

1   **surface apoproteins**

2   **apoproteins - A, C & E + other transmembrane, & regulatory proteins for transport of internal materials**

3   **cholesterol - free on the surface - esterified inside, small amounts in the membrane**

4   **phospholipid membrane layer - in VLDL & Chylomicorns - almost devoid of protein**

5   **TGAs + FFAs**

TGAs
FFAs

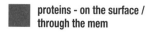
proteins - on the surface / through the mem

cholesterol - outside
cholestrylester - inside

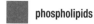
phospholipids

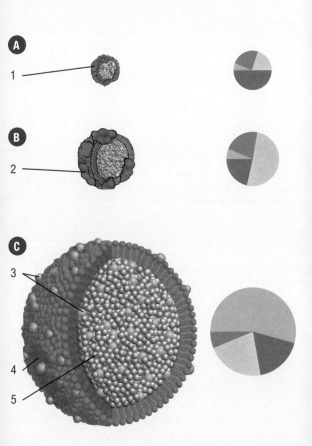

Lipoprotein pathways

Cholesterol & fats are transported from the GIT, to the liver via chylomicrons, through the SI lacteals.

The liver exports LDLs as the major supply of fats & cholesterol for tissue use.

Specific tissue receptors absorb the apoproteins & contents of the LDLs, according to needs; converting LDLs → HDLs

HDLs are returned to the liver - REVERSE TRANSPORT & are made into bile salts.

Bile salts are secreted into the duodenum - 95% are resorbed in the terminal ileum, recycling the cholesterol.

Excess cholesterol & fats stay in the LDLs, but cannot be absorbed by most Ts because of the lack of apoproteins.

LDLs are converted to VLDLs, lacking surface proteins.

VLDLs can only be absorbed by adipose T & resident BV macrophages.

Macrophages containing excessive fats & cholesterol are converted to foam cells.

Foam cells undermine the structure of the vascular endothelium & lead to atheromatous plaque formation.

1. **GIT → liver of emulsified fats & cholesterol - CHYLOMICRONS**
2. **export of LDLS**
3. **LDLs to Tissues - muscle & AT absorb the largest amounts**
4. **HDLs remain & return to the liver**
5. **bile salts - secretion & resorption in the GIT**
6. **excess cholesterol is moved from HDLs & LDLs to VLDLs via CETP**
7. **VLDLs absorbed from BVs to macrophages which become foam cells**

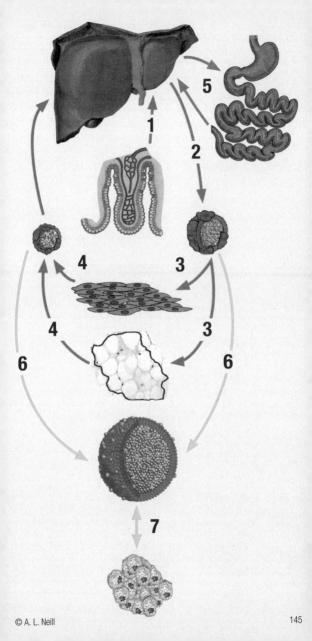

Melatonin synthesis

Melatonin is primarily synthesised in the pineal gland. It may also be synthesised in other organs - in particular the gonads - where it acts as a powerful antioxidant. It regulates the diurnal rhythm, in mammals. The pathway is similar to that of serotonin & dopamine. These Hs are all derived from the AA tryptophan.

The rate limiting step is the degradation of the cAMP-dependent protein kinase A (PKA) **11E**, in daylight.

PKA phosphorylates the penultimate enzyme, the arylalkylamine N-acetyltransferase (NAT) **3E**, the last step in the pathway & not affecting the earlier synthesis of serotonin (3).

Noradrenergic stimulation via the receptors (28) of the pinealocyte (26) stops at daylight & restarts

again in the evening, which is called the dim-light melatonin onset (DLMO).

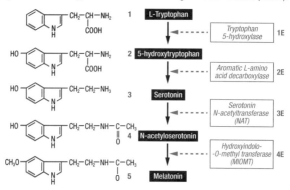

10E adenalate cyclase
11E protein kinase A
20 retina
21 suprachiasmatic nucleus
22 PVN
23 upper thoracic SC segment
24 intermediolateral cell column
25 superior cervical ganglion
26 pinealocyte
27 capillary
28 adrenergic receptors - a = α b = β

© A. L. Neill

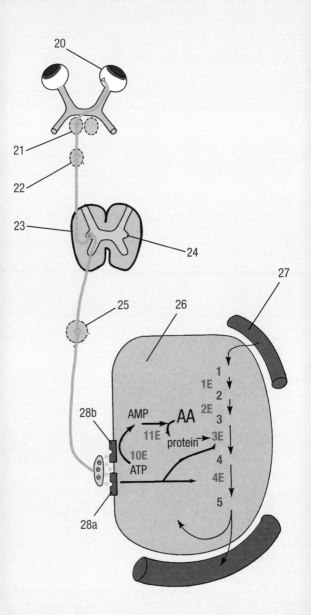

© A. L. Neill

Melatonin -
Pineal - Hypothalamic - Pituitary loop

Melatonin stimulated via nocturnal noradrenergic stimulation (related to UV levels) is produced by the pineal gland (1), and is one of the higher centres which influences the hypothalamus (2). By establishing the body's circadian rhythm, the H secretions of the other major endocrine organs are also affected.

1 **Melatonin (from the pineal gland) regulates the body clock**

2 **↑ melatonin causes ↑ RFs (from the hypothalamus)**

3 **which stimulates GH & ACTH (from the ant. pit.)**

4 **releasing IGF (from the liver) (*IGF= insulin like growth factor*)**

5 **releasing Cortisol (from the adrenal)**

6 **releasing DHEA (from the adrenal)**

7 **↑ Cortisol inhibits - ACTH & GH release from the ant. pit.**

8 **↑ Cortisol inhibits the RFs from the hypothalamus**

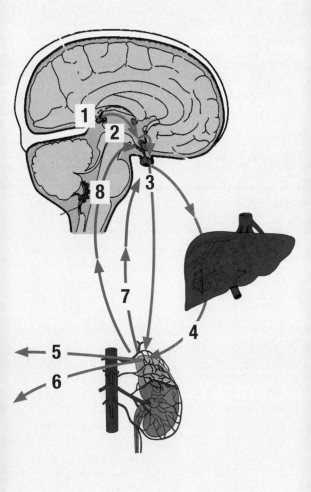

Parathyroid Hormone (PTH)

Calcium Phosphate regulation - normal

PTH is the main H controlling the B[Ca] & [PO] levels. With ↑ PO levels PTH ↑ & may result in elimination of Ca from the body. Both ions are in balance - Ca X PO = Z.

Because of Ca's role in N transmission & muscle contraction the B[Ca] must be very tightly controlled, even at the cost of bone strength.

Both Ca & PO need Vita C & D for adequate absorption, re-sorption from the kidney & maintenance of serum levels.

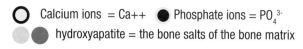

○ Calcium ions = Ca++ ● Phosphate ions = PO_4^{3-}

hydroxyapatite = the bone salts of the bone matrix

1. parathyroid glands
2. thyroid gland
3. PH pathway
4. Ca & PO normally diffuse across the renal tubules
5. PH – causes Ca to be reabsorbed but inhibits PO
6. remaining Ca & PO lost in the urine
7. bone matrix + hydroxyapatite – OCs ↑
8. Vitamin C + acidity ↑
9. OCs
10. Normally bone formation (bf)= resorption (bs) bf>bs growth / bf<bs OP
11. OB (laying down bone)
12. B-AP ↑ with bone formation
13. S(Ca) ↓ S(PO) ↓ – move into bone
14. blood pH – acidity favours blood Ca ↑ (out of bone) – alkalinity favours blood Ca ↓ & PO ↓ (into bone)
15. GIT secretions – including bile / stomach acid / pancreatic enzymes facilitate
16. Vitamin D to absorb Ca & PO across the gut
17. Cortisol opposes the action of Vitamin D
18. Ca / PO balance directly affects the PH levels – both high levels of Ca or PO ↓ PH – low levels of Ca ↑ PH

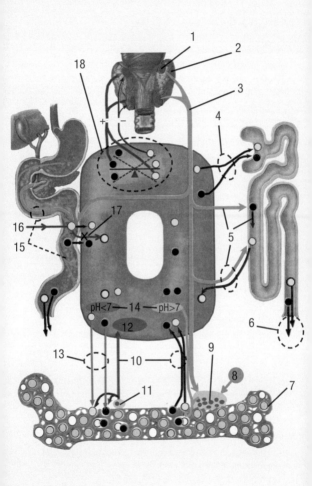

pH<7 — 14 — pH>7

Parathyroid Hormone (PTH)

Calcium Phosphate regulation -
HYPERPARATHYROIDISM

PTH is the main H controlling the B[Ca] & [PO] levels. With ↑ PO levels PTH ↑ & may result in elimination of Ca from the body. Both ions are in balance - Ca X PO = Z. This occurs in hyperparathyroidism.

Excessive PTH levels result in Osteitis Fibrosa Cystica.

Bone density becomes irregular with strong bone trabeculae being replaced by weaker fibrous T & cysts.

Pathological #s occur; Kidney stones may develop along with ↑ nausea & anorexia.

⚪ Calcium ions = Ca++   ⚫ Phosphate ions = PO_4^{3-}

  hydroxyapatite = the bone salts of the bone matrix

1   parathyroid glands with hyperparathyroidism due to:
    a = adenoma – 80% / b = clear cell hyperplasia – 10%
    / c = chief cell hyperplasia – 8% / d = carcinoma of the
    parathyroid gland – 2%
2   thyroid gland
3   PTH pathway – ↑ due to hyperparathyroidism & causing
4   ↑ serum levels of Ca – but low PO levels
5   ↑ levels of Ca are excreted via the kidney due to the
        high serum levels
6   ↑ PO levels are excreted via the kidney because
        resorption is blocked via the PTH
Leading to the formation of renal stones (7)
8   PTH – ↑ OCs to resorb bone causing
9   bone cysts ("brown" tumours) – pathological #s
10 irregular bone density develops – partic subperiosteal
    resorption & fibrous replacement from irregular OC
    stimulation & irregular OB stimulation
11 OB – laying down additional bone in response to the
    resorption & ↑ serum Ca
12 B-AP ↑ with bone formation
13 PTH causes ↑ Ca & PO absorption from the GIT so ...
14   ↑ movement to the bone

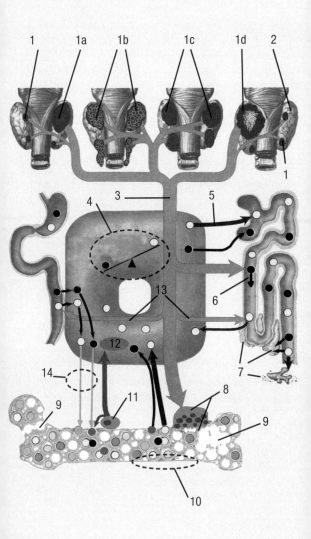

Parathyroid Hormone (PTH)

Calcium Phosphate regulation -
HYPOPARATHYROIDISM

PTH is the main H controlling the B[Ca] & [PO] levels. The commonest reason for hypoparathyroidism is iatrogenic - the accidental removal or damage during thyroid surgery. Other causes are congenital absence or chemical shutdown.

B[PO] ↑ with the absence or decrease of PTH. OCs are inhibited & Ca is not mobilized from bone.

However the bone continues to be laid down at the normal rate.

○   Calcium ions = Ca++   ● Phosphate ions = PO_4^{3-}

    hydroxyapatite = the bone salts of the bone matrix

1. **parathyroid glands absent due to surgery (a) or other rare causes (b) eg congenital.**
2. **Ca – PO balance – PO ↑ and Ca reduced**
3. **PTH pathway – absent due to lack of glands**
   4. **Ca absorption from the GIT ↓ – no PTH**
   5. **Ca absorption from the GIT ↓ binds to the ↑ PO**
6. **urine Ca ↓ because of the low serum levels**
7. **urine PO ↓ it is actively resorbed from the kidneys no PTH to block it**
8. **OCs ↓ Ca & PO not mobilized and bone turnover is ↓ no PTH**
9. **OBs continue unaffected by the loss of PTH – laying down new bone**
10. **bone density ↑**
11. **Alkaline phosphatase unaffected**

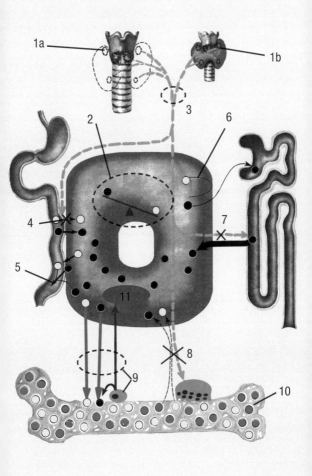

Polypeptides / Proteins - general

Formation of a polypeptide (PP)

A PP is a chain of AAs joined together by peptide bonds, b/n C atoms & either the amide or carboxyl groups (1). The amide end group is the N terminus (2) & the carboxyl group the C terminus (3). AAs may be added to either end.

Each AA has a distinct side chain (R) which may be hydrophilic (4) or hydrophobic (5). With increasing PP length the chain folds to move the hydrophobic AAs (5) internally away from the hydrophilic intracellular environment, leaving the hydrophilic AAs on the outer surface.

A chain > 50AAs is a Protein, but there is a lot of overlap b/n these 2 terms. *see also Amino Acids (AA)*

1	**Carbon atoms**
2	**N terminus**
3	**C terminus**
4	**R side chain - hydrophilic**
5	**R side chain - hydrophobic**

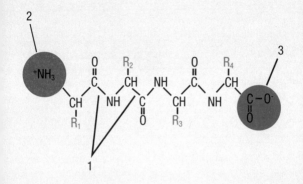

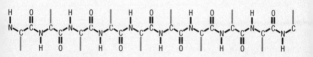

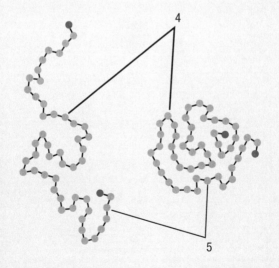

Polypeptides / Proteins - folding

Schema of protein folding formation

Protein folding is the process by which a proteins assumes its 3D bioactive shape from a random coil. Proteins begin as AAs joined together with peptide bonds to form PP chains *1° structure* (1). The AAs then interact & form a well-defined 3D folded state - **the Native State**, which is determined by: the AA sequence, mRNA codon, presence of chaperones & external conditions. The folding places hydrophobic sequences internally protecting them from the watery environment, & the hydrophilic sequences externally. It is highly organized but may take several pathways going from a simple AA chain to *2° folding* (2)- formation of α helices & β pleated sheets which combine in ever increasing complexities *3° folding* (3) & may combine then with other protein subunits ± other ions / sugars etc to become fully operative proteins *4° folding* (4).

Correct folding is needed for protein functionality. Consistent mis-folding (5) may produce inactive proteins, amyloidosis / allergies / random toxicities, which can occur at any stage in this process.

1. *1° structure* of AA chain
2. *2° folding* = natural 3D structure = the native state
3. *3° folding* - repeated protein patterns to fill in and build the protein
4. *4° folding* - protein subunit additions added to change or modify the protein shape & activate it - completed protein eg. an enzyme / H/ ECM - large amounts will build up in the cell & render it useless
5. mis-folding formation of inactive or pathological protein material

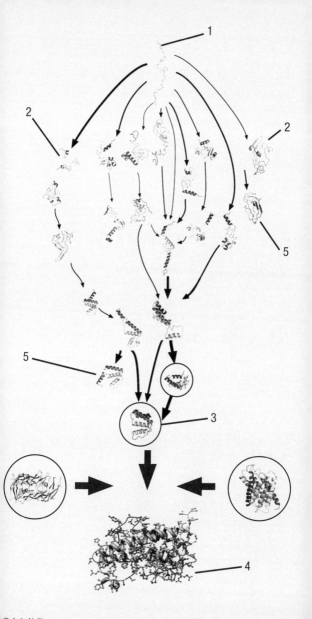

Polypeptides / Proteins - filler structures

α *helix*

The α helix is a R-Handed coil of AAs in which every N-H group **(1)** of one AA binds to the C=O group of the AA 4 residues earlier **(2)** with H bonds **(3)** - forming a consistent 13 AA coil, with the AA side chains pointing out of the spiral **(4)**. It is one of the 2 structures found in 2° protein folding.

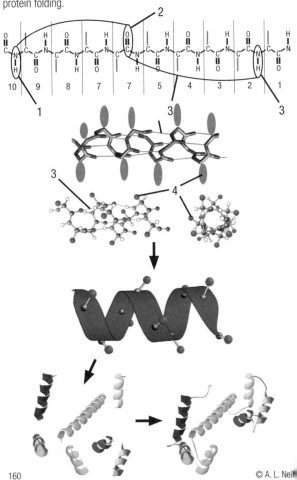

© A. L. Neil

β pleated sheets

A The β pleated sheet is a structure of 20 protein folding where small (< 6) PP chains line up & form **H bonds** through **N-H groups** of one AA with the **C=O groups** of another PP chain on the opposite line. They may be parallel **(1)** or anti-parallel **(2)** in that their carboxyl ends may face or oppose each other.

B This is repeated over 6 chains and results in a pleated appearance with the different radical groups (R) **(3)** of the AAs facing outwards.

C The different linkages in the β sheets are H bonds **(4)** b/n them & peptide bonds **(5)** along the PP chain the backbone of the β sheets.

D The peptide backbone is represented when illustrated in molecule modeling by thick ribbons of peptide chains **(6)**. **E**

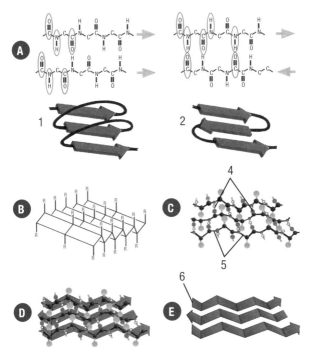

Vitamin A AKA Retinol AKA Retinal / Retinoic Acid*

FAT SOLUBLE VITAMIN

3 active forms of Vita A in the body :

1 - pro- vitamin A AKA ß carotene which can easily be converted to Vita A as needed, by the liver.

2 - retinoids, & - "pre-formed" Vita A.

3 - 3D form of Vitamin A

Benefits	Recommended amount (daily RDA or daily AI)	Deficiency	Good food sources
↑ night vision ↓ cataract formation ↑ skin texture / healing ↑ cancers partic prostate/ respiratory ß carotenoids act as antioxidants	M: 900 mcg (3,000 IU) W: 700 mcg (2,333 IU) **note narrow range of toxicity**	night-blindness dry thin skin	**Sources of retinoids:** beef, liver, eggs, shrimp, fish, fortified milk, cheese, **Sources of ß carotene:** sweet potatoes, carrots, pumpkins, squash, spinach, mangoes, turnip greens
Functions	**Upper limit per day**	**Toxicity**	**Storage sites**
precursor to retinal - the prosthetic group to all 4 light absorbing pigments in the eye regulating gene expression to maintain epithelia ↑ osteoclast / ↓ osteoblasts- hence ↑ bone mobility ↑ B[Ca]	3,000 mcg (about 10,000 IU in adults - 1500IU in children)	children are partic susceptible carotenes - are not toxic	Liver 80% Fats 10-20% Lung 3-5% Kidneys 1-3%

* While these terms are used interchangably the structures vary - but collectively they make up *Vita A*

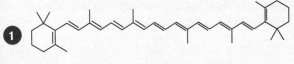

1

2 R

R = CH$_2$OH = retinol = vitamin A

R = CHO = retinal

R = COOH = retinoic acid = tretinoin

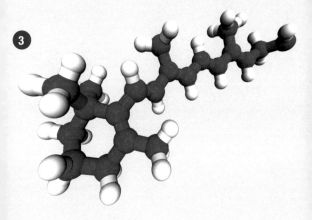

3

Hypervitaminosis A

Toxicity of Vitamin A - a fat soluble vitamin

Vita A competes with the other fat soluble Vitas D, E & K, for absorption. It has a direct effect on Vita D metabolism & competes with it by mobilizing bone. This is particularly relevant in children who are very sensitive to Hypervitaminosis A. Chronic long term hypervitaminosis A has been associated with ↑ of cancers particularly prostate and respiratory cancers.

Reduction in Vita A consumption, & ↑ Vita E corrects the condition.

	Acute / short term	Chronic / long terms
Bone changes due to ↑ Ca mobilization ↓ osteoclast activity ↑ osteoblast activity ↑ bone softening	bone / head pain	bone / head pain ↑ intracranial P pathological # OP **calcification of Ts including heart valves (in children)** **craniotabes (in children)** **premature epiphyseal plate closure (in children)**
Consciousness changes	dizziness drowsiness irritability	
GIT changes	anorexia nausea / vomiting	gastric mucosal calcinosis liver damage **poor weight gain (in children)**
Skin / adnexae changes due to ↓ expression of precursor for maintenance of the epithelia ↑ serum [Carotenoids]	discoloration of the skin (aurantiasis cutis) ↑ sun damage uremic pruritus	chelosis hair loss / cracked nails oily skin & hair (seborrhea)
Vision changes due to changes in the [visual pigment] changes in skull formation	photophobia	blurred vision diplopia (in children)

Notes

Vitamin B1 AKA Thiamin AKA Thiamine AKA Thio - vitamine / Sulphur containing vitamin

WATER SOLUBLE VITAMIN
C12H17CIN4OS-

Benefits	Recommended amount (daily RDA or daily AI)	Deficiency	Good food sources
Helps convert food into E particularly - in N conduction & cardiac muscle	M: 1.2 mg, W: 1.1 mg	beriberi - not common in dev. countries found in alcoholics. Kosakovs & Wernicke's syndrome SS - fatigue, N damage, psychosis & weakness then amnesia, confabulation & irreversible dementia,	Pork chops, ham, soymilk, watermelons, acorn squash Most nutritious/ "enriched" foods have some thiamin
Functions	**Upper limit per day**	**Interesting facts**	**Storage sites**
coenzyme - in cellular respiration thiamin pyrophosphate (TPP) converting pyruvate to acetyl CoA used in the synthesis of acetylcholine & GABA & other neurotransmitters	NOT KNOWN easily excreted	first called aneurin as it caused neurological effects when not present in the diet necessary. inh first stage of alcohol fermentation	25-30mg stored in muscle, brain, liver & kidneys

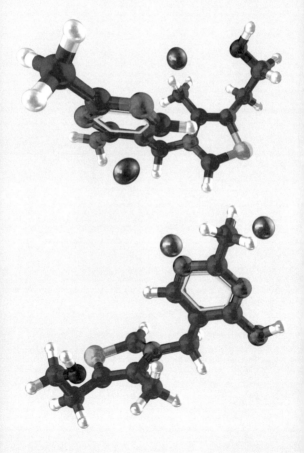

Vitamin B2 AKA Riboflavin

WATER SOLUBLE VITAMIN
C17H20N4O6-

Benefits	Recommended amount (daily RDA or daily AI)	Deficiency	Good food sources
Helps convert food into E Needed for healthy skin, hair, RBCs, & brain	M: 1.3 mg, W: 1.1 mg	damage to eyes, mouth, and genitals, ariboflavinosis ss - cheilosis, high sensitivity to sunlight, glossitis, seborrheic dermatitis, pharyngitis, inflammation of the mms including labia & scrotum	Milk, yoghurt, cheese, whole & enriched grains & cereals, liver
Functions	**Upper limit per day**	**Interesting facts**	**Storage**
prosthetic group of flavoprotein enzymes, e.g., flavin adenine dinucleotide (FAD) used in cellular respiration ß oxidation, FFA oxidation	NOT KNOWN easily excreted	this Vita is destroyed by exposure to sunlight it has a distinctive YELLOW COLOUR which colours urine yellow	

1 riboflavin

   H = reduced form of riboflavin

2 R group = the enzyme attached which is using the riboflavin / or possibly PO4 attached when it is present as a salt

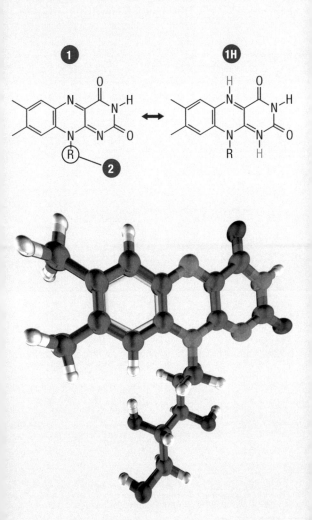

Vitamin B3 AKA Niacin AKA Nicotinic acid

WATER SOLUBLE VITAMIN
C6H5NO2

Benefits	Recommended amount (daily RDA or daily AI)	Deficiency	Good food sources
Helps convert food into E, Essential for healthy skin, GIT function, brain function, & NS. Decreases the risk of cardiovascular disease	M: 16 mg, W: 14 mg	mild - slow metabolism, intolerance to cold, digestive problems, insomnia & weakness	Meat, poultry, fish, fortified & whole grains, mushrooms, potatoes, nuts & legumes
		severe - Pellegra	common in most foods & enriched foods
		SS include aggression, confusion, dementia, dermatitis, diarrhoea, & death	
Functions	**Upper limit per day**	**Toxicity**	**Interesting fact**
Niacin is composed of 2 structures: nicotinic acid & nicotinamide, which form two co-enzymes NAD & NADP. Both involved in E transfer in the metabolism of glucose, FFAs & alcohol. NAD carries hydrogens & their electrons during metabolic reactions, the citric acid cycle & the electron transport chain. NADP is a co-enzyme in lipid & nucleic acid synthesis.	35 mg	flushing, dermatitis, pruritis, liver damage, maculopathy, peptic ulcers,	Niacin can be made by the body from tryptophan, + Vita B6 + Vita B2 + iron.

1 **niacin**

2 **synthesis from tryptophan**

    2a = tryptophan

    2b = serotonin

    2c = melatonin

    2d = niacin

3 **niacin 3D**

1

2a

2b

2c

2d

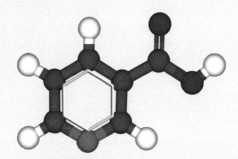

Vitamin B6 AKA Pyridoxine AKA Pyridoxal AKA Pyridoxamine

WATER SOLUBLE VITAMIN
C8H11NO3

Benefits	Recommended amount (daily RDA or daily AI)	Deficiency	Good food sources
↓ homocysteine ↓ the risk of heart disease ↓ PMS symptoms ↓ nausea ↑ mental alertness ↑ macula preservation	M: 1.7 mg, W: 1.5 mg	anaemia	Beans, cereals, vegetables, liver, meat, and eggs. common in most foods & enriched foods
Functions	**Upper limit per day**	**Toxicity**	**Storage**
used in conjunction with other B Vitas as a coenzyme in many reactions	200 mg	irreversible neurotoxicity - from excessive supplements severe difficulty in walking, peripheral anaesthesia mild : pain & numbness of the extremities.	liver

1 **pyridoxine 2D structure**
2 **pyridoxine as a phosphate - rotated to show 3D structure**

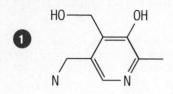

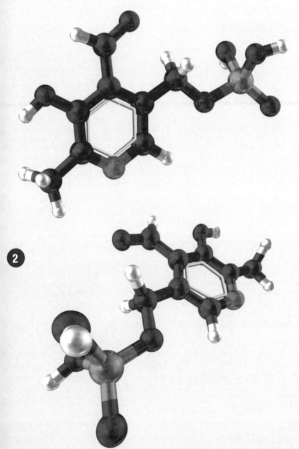

Vitamin B7 AKA Biotin AKA Vitamin H AKA Coenzyme R

WATER SOLUBLE VITAMIN
C10H16N2O3S

Benefits	Recommended amount (daily RDA or daily AI)	Deficiency	Good food sources
↓ homocysteine ↓ the risk of heart disease ↓ PMS symptoms ↓ nausea ↑ mental alertness ↑ macula preservation ↑ hair nails & skin	not known ~	caused by binding to egg whites, poor diet, intestinal malabsorption rare otherwise ss rashes, alopecia, anaemia, seborrhoeic dermatitis, susceptibility to fungal Ins, generalized pains severe anorexia depression, lethargy, weakness	mostly from the bacteria in the GIT also most foods associated with the other Vita Bs dragon fruit, egg yolk
Functions used as a coenzyme involved in the synthesis of FFAs, glucose, isoleucine & valine coenzyme for the carboxylase enzymes	**Upper limit per day** not known	**Toxicity** irreversible neurotoxicity - from excessive supplements severe: difficulty in walking, peripheral anaesthesia mild: pain & numbness of the extremities.	**Interesting facts** used in assays - due to the strong bond it forms - eg with egg white protein avidin

1 **Biotin 2D structure**
2 **Biotin 3D structure**

1

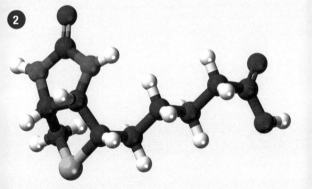

2

175

Vitamin B9 AKA Folic acid AKA Folate AKA Vitamin M AKA Vitamin Bc

WATER SOLUBLE VITAMIN
C19H19N7O6

Benefits	Recommended amount (daily RDA or daily AI)	Deficiency	Good food sources
↑ RBCs prevents birth defects	M:1mg W: 1mg pregnant W 1.4mg ~	anaemia, possible birth defects in pregnant W note it masks Vita B12 deficiency and this can lead to permanent neurological deficit	mostly from vegetables but destroyed by cooking in enriched breads - min requirement bc of demands by pregnant women
Functions	**Upper limit per day**	**Toxicity**	
used as a coenzyme involved in the synthesis purines & pyrimidines	not known	not stored easily excreted supplemental OD only form of toxicity nausea, bloating, sleep disturbances, SOB, rash	

1   folic acid - 2D structure
2   folic acid - 3D structure
3   movement of the 3D folic acid molecule

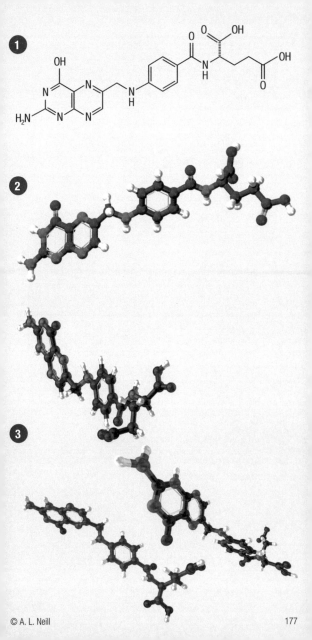

Vitamin B12 AKA Cobalamin

WATER SOLUBLE VITAMIN largest & most complex
C63H88CoN14O14P

Benefits	Recommended amount (daily RDA or daily AI)	Deficiency	Good food sources
essential for blood, N health & muscle contraction	none identified difficult to absorb partic for vegans & the elderly	pernicious anaemia rash ? peripheral neuropathy weakness & loss of balance. ↑ homocysteine	produced by bacteria needs "intrinsic factor" from stomach parietal cells for absorption can only e made artificially from bacteria

Functions	Upper limit per day	Storage	Interesting facts
used as a coenzyme involved in the synthesis DNA, FFAs & protein essential for RBCs	not known	liver can store for up to 3 yrs worth	contains Cobalt which is at the base of the CORRIN ring converts to **cyancobalamin** which metabolised leaves cyanide ion behind

1 **cobalamin - line 2D structure**
   a = R at the active site = -OH / -CN / -Me
   c = corrin ring
   n = nucleotide loop
2 **cyancobalamin - 2D structure**
   c = R = -CN
3 **cobalamin 2D molecule showing the surrounding corrin ring**
4 **cobalamin 3D structure**

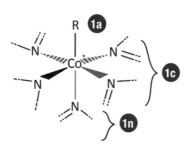

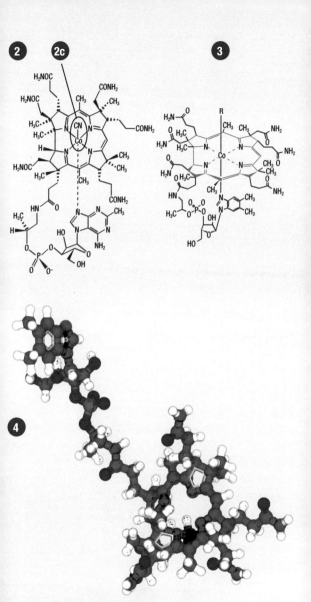

© A. L. Neill

Vitamin "B- like substances"

WATER SOLUBLE VITAMINs

Many substances have been called Vita Bs in the past. They are a collection of substances found in whole unprocessed foods - generally together. If through processing they are leached out they are often replaced - "enriching" the food.

They have no structural similarities, but they are essential for life, and most act as co-enzymes for essential reactions. While most are produced from plants - some com from meat - GI bacteria.

They have a plethora of names because of the way they were discovered and this can be confusing. Most are not stored & do not show toxicity except when there is a supplement OD.

Below is a list of all the other "Vita Bs". They are here for completeness

Vitamin B4:   Adenine (a nucleobase); or Choline which is synthesised in the body but in small amounts and supplemented form the diet. It is now considered as an essential dietary nutrient.

Vitamin B8:   adenosine monophosphate (AMP) AKA adenylic acid. inositol

Vitamin B10 / Bx: pABA or PABA, a chemical component of folate. It is used as a UV -blocking sunscreen cream applied to the skin.

Vitamin B11:   pteryl-hepta-glutamic acid—chick growth factor, another form of folic acid essential for N growth AKA Vitamin Bc-conjugate which was PHGA.

Vitamin B13:   orotic acid

Vitamin B15:   pangamate, no longer available as it is unsafe .

Vitamin B16:   DMG which is part of the Citric acid (or Kreb's) cycle.

Vitamin B17:   nitrilosides found in a number of seeds, sprouts, beans, tubers, and grains.

Vitamin B20 / Bf / Bm / BT: Carnitine. (also Vita B4)

Vitamin Bv: a type of Vita B6

Vitamin Bw: a type of Biotin.

Vitamin B4

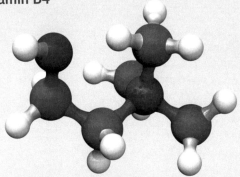

Vitamin B8

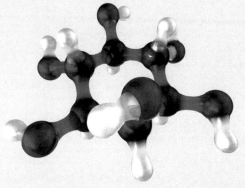

Vitamin B10

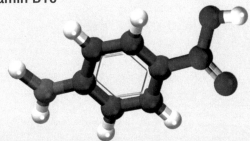

Vitamin C AKA Ascorbic acid AKA Ascorbate

WATER SOLUBLE VITAMIN
$C_6H_6O_6$

Benefits	Recommended amount (daily RDA or daily AI)	Deficiency	Good food sources
possible cancer protection possible cataract protection ↑ collagen ↑ healing involved in neurotransmitter synthesis serotonin & noradrenalin antioxidant bolsters the immune system	M: 90 mg, W: 75 mg smokers: + 35 mg	scurvy it is not known how much Vita C is stored	Fruits & fruit juices (especially citrus), potatoes, broccoli, bell peppers, spinach, strawberries, tomatoes, Brussels sprouts
Functions	**Upper limit per day**	**Toxicity**	**Interesting facts**
used as a coenzyme involved in the synthesis collagen	2,000 mg although many take more than this animals frequently take 10X-20X more than this	none known humans are able to recycle Vita C	most animals synthesize this molecule used as a preservative

1 ascorbate - 2D structure ascorbic acid (reduced form)
   → dehydroascorbic acid (oxidized form)
2 ascorbate - 3D structure

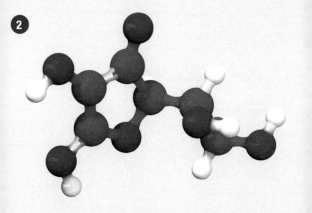

Vitamin Ds

FAT SOLUBLE VITAMINs (Vitamers)

Several active forms of Vita D in the body all secosteroids i.e. steroids with a broken ring :

D1 AKA Ergocalciferal

D2 AKA Ergocalciferal - from ergosterol AKA calciferal

D3 AKA Cholecalciferal from 7-dehydrocholesterol in the skin AKA calciferal

D4 AKA 22-dihydroergocalciferal

D5 AKA Sitocalciferal from 7-dehydrocholesterol in the skin -

Vitamins D2 & D3 are collectively referred to as calciferol most active & important of the Vita Ds. Vita D refers to D2 + D3 forms of the vitamin.

Benefits	Recommended amount (daily RDA or daily AI)	Deficiency	Good sources
acts as a H to maintain B[Ca] & B[PO4] & maintains bone density along with PTH. other ions absorbed are iron, magnesium & zinc	31–50yo: 5 mcg (200 IU)	Osteomalacia	sunlight supplements the dietary requirements
used to prevent pathological #s used to activate the immune system & neuromuscular function	51–70yo: 10 mcg (400 IU) 71+: 15 mcg (600 IU)	Rickets - in children	fortified milk or margarine, fortified cereals, fatty fish
	needs increase with age - & lack of sun exposure		note plants do not make Vita D only precursors
Functions	**Upper limit per day**	**Toxicity**	**Storage Sites**
active Vita D works with PTH Calcitonin to regulate Ca & Po4 levels	50 mcg (2,000 IU)	calcification in soft Ts	Liver- stored as the pro-H
		mental retardation in children	calcidiol - inactive - converted in the kidney to active form calciferol
			also found in the skin & AT

1 **ergosterol a steroid converted to**
2 **D2 in fungi a secosteroid**
3 **7-dehydrocholesterol a steroid converted to**
4 **D3 in the skin of animals a secosteroid**
5 **conversion via UV in sunlight**
6 **broken steroid ring**

① ⑤ ② C₂H ⑥ ③ ⑤ ④ C₂H

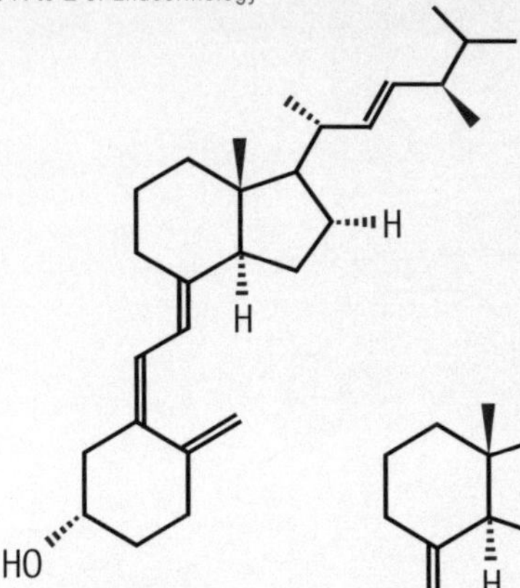

Vita D2

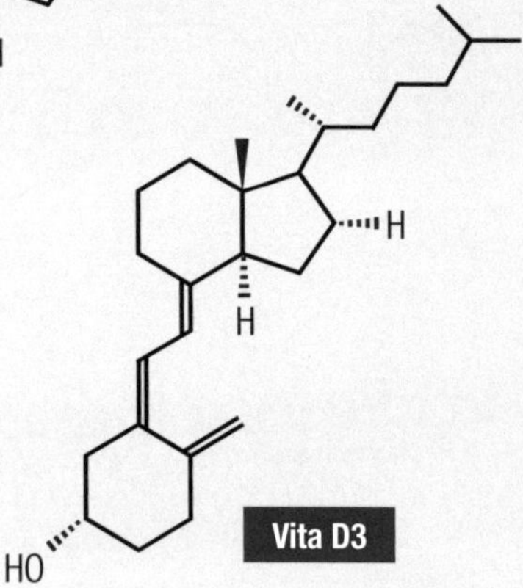

Vita D3

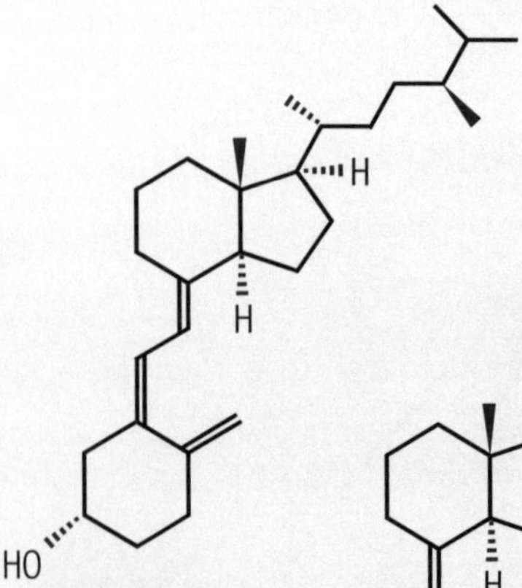

Vita D4

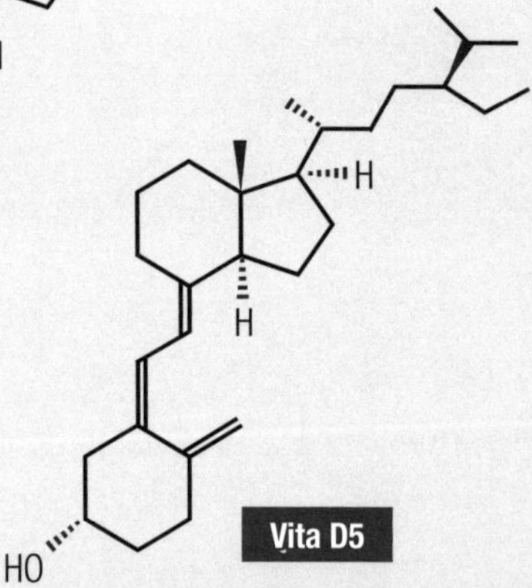

Vita D5

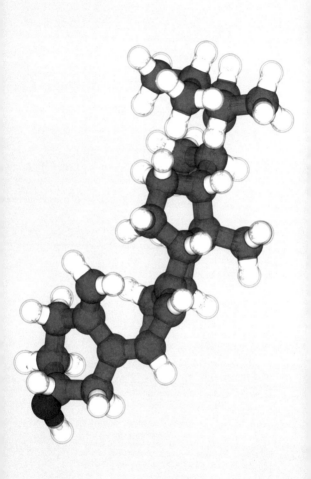

Vitamin Ds - metabolism

Schema of activation & synthesis via the liver, kidney & skin
Calcitriol AKA (1,25(OH)$_2$D) AKA 1, 25 -dihyroxycholcalciferol
- the active form of Vita D

Vitamin D3 is synthesizes in the skin from cholesterol →
7-dehydrocholesterol, via UV light. The liver converts D3 into an inactive
form Calcidiol, where it binds to a binding globulin & is transported
to the kidney for final activation, and conversion to the active form
Calciterol. This conversion is mediated by ↑ PTH ↓ Ca & ↓ PO4.

Calciterol is transported by a binding globulin in the B to the target
organs.

Depending upon the B[Ca] the parathyroid gland ↑ PTH which regulates
how much Vita D is synthesized in the skin &/ or how much Vita D
is actively absorbed in the GI tract, as well as regulating Ca & PO4
absorption.

1 the UV in sunlight forms Vita D3
2 transported down to the liver - deactivated to calcidiol -
   inactive form of Vita D
3 transported to the kidney for activation depending upon
   the B[Ca]/[PO4]
4 dietary intake of Vita D generally D2 / D3
   absorbed via the SI / also Ca & other ions absorbed via
   the SI
5 transported to the liver
6 ↓ B[Ca] or ↓ [PO4] causes PTH ↑
   which activates Vita D in the kidney
   facilitating additional GIT absorption of Ca /PO4
   additional Vita D synthesis
   & Ca mobilization from the bone
7 activated Vita D maintains bone mineralization & Ca
   absorption

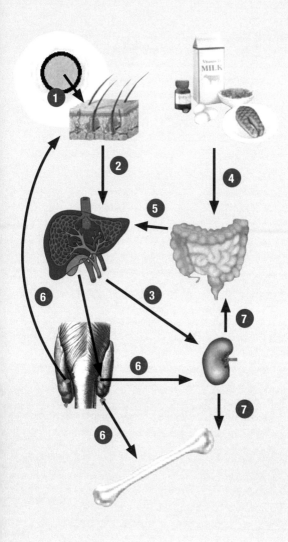

Hypovitaminosis D - Osteomalacia / Rickets

Osteomalacia (OM) is due to a defect in bone matrix mineralisation UNDERMINERALIZATION, due to ↓ serum Ca (1). The disease is called Rickets when it presents in children or immature growing bones.

Causes of which are:
- *lack of Vitamin D - hypovitaminosis, disturbance in the absorption of Vitamin D (2) associated with disturbances in fat absorption due to GB, pancreatic deficiencies - sprue malabsorption or its metabolism via the liver*
- *inadequate sunlight - partic UV to allow the formation of Vitamin D (3)*
- *↑ dietary PO4 or phytates (4) which inhibits Ca absorption across the GIT (5) serum levels of Ca X PO4 = K*
- *↑ demands for Ca as in pregnancy or lactation (6) - or excessive sweating*
- *↓ re-absorption of Ca from the kidney in the distal convoluted tubules (7).*

↑ serum Ca - causes 2º parathyroid hyperplasia (8) & ↑ PTH levels (9) via feedback (10) hence PO4 reabsorption is ↓ across the renal tubules (11); maintaining the low serum levels of both Ca & PO4 (12) Ca & PO4 is mobilized from the bone – via the OCs (13) but does not come out of the blood (14) – even though the OBs (15) are stimulated by the weak bone to form more & more bone. Hence the bone is poorly formed & undermineralized (16) – Leading to irregular lucent areas of bone – (17) Looser's lines or bodies AKA pseudofractures AKA Milkman's syndrome & moth-eaten EPs in immature bones (18). The turnover of the bone is ↑ reflected in the ↑ serum levels of AP. OBs lay down excessive osteoid T seams beneath the periosteum (19) and this leads to ↑ BVs (20) & fibrous T in the LB – flattening & broadening these bones in the adult & bending them in the child.

Typical features are similar to those of Paget's disease:

- Flat occiput, frontal bossing & square head
- Overgrowth of cartilage at costochondral junctions
- Pigeon chest
- Harrison's sulcus
- Lumbar lordosis
- Leg bowing
- Pathological #s particularly the VBs & NOF
- ↑ in CO and metabolism in general

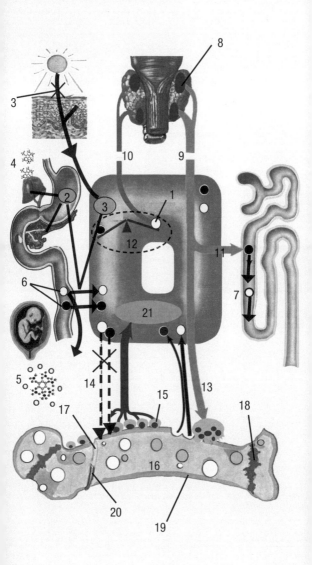

Vitamin E AKA Tocopherol AKA α-Tocopherol

FAT SOLUBLE VITAMIN
Found in 2 major forms
1 Tocopherols
2 Tocotrienals
3 3D representation of Vita E

Benefits	Recommended amount (daily RDA or daily AI)	Deficiency	Good food sources
an antioxidant, preventing oxidative damage	M: 15 mg, W: 15 mg (15 mg = about 22 IU from natural sources of Vita E & 33 IU from synthetic Vita E)	anaemia retinal damage	nuts, spinach vegetable oils,
protects Vita A & certain lipids from damage			
Vita E may help prevent Alzheimer's disease & protect against prostate cancer			
Functions	**Upper limit (UL) per day**	**Toxicity**	**Interesting facts**
preserves cms	1,000 mg (nearly 1,500 IU natural Vita E; 2,200 IU synthetic)	competes with Vita K for absorption - hence bleeding problems may develop	no studies have confirmed properties purported for this Vita - i.e. no protection from cancer / no increase in fertility or virility / no decrease in aging or improved skin

1

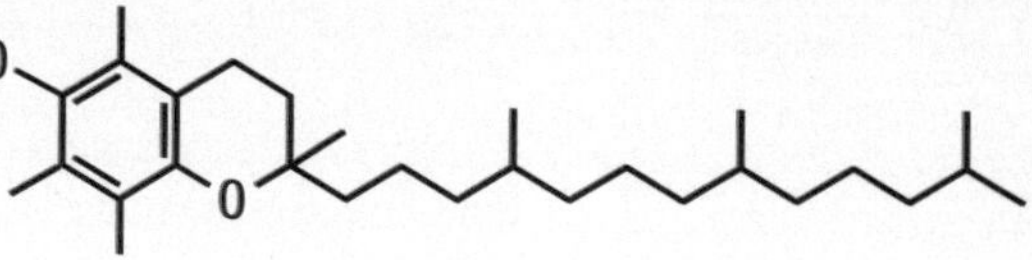

2

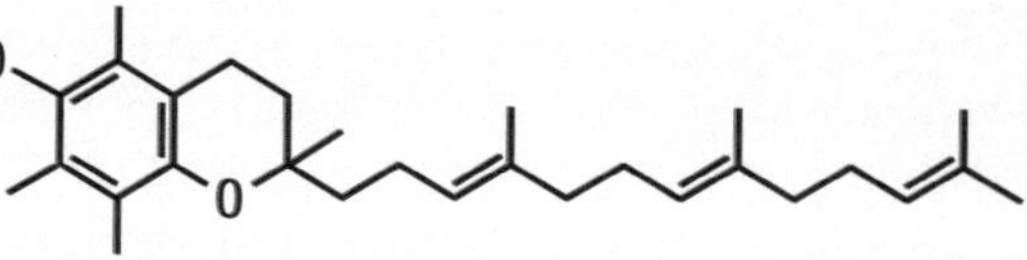

3

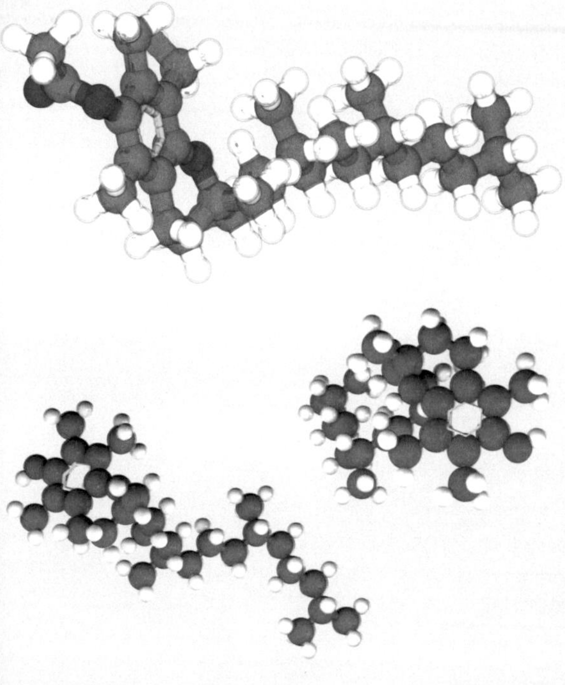

Vitamin K

FAT SOLUBLE VITAMIN
Found in 2 forms K1 - phylloquinone (1) K2 - menadione (2)
the repeating units (isoprenoid in K2) may vary b/n 1-5 in
each case

Benefits	Recommended amount (daily RDA* or daily AI**)	Deficiency	Good food sources
Activates proteins & Ca essential to blood clotting May help prevent #	M: 120 mcg, W: 90 mcg	weakened bones	Cabbage, liver, eggs, milk, spinach, broccoli, sprouts, kale, collards, & other green vegetables GI bacteria
Functions needed for the synthesis of clotting factors needed for the binding of Ca to bone in some mineralization	**Upper limit (UL) per day** not known	**Toxicity** not known	**Storage sites** AT in the body

1

2

ENDOCRINE ORGANS AND THEIR HORMONES

Endocrine Organs	Main Hormones Secreted	Target Organ	Main Endocrine Functions
Adipose Tissue	ADIPOKINES RESISTIN	Whole Body	↑ metabolism ↑ appetite & IR pro-If
	ADIPONECTIN LEPTIN		↓ appetite suppressant & IR anti-IF
Adrenal Cortex	GLUCOCORTICOIDS corticosterone, cortisol MINERCORTICOIDS aldosterone	Kidney Whole Body	↑ B [glucose] ↑ reabsorption of Na+ & excretion of K+ anti-IF
	SEX Hs androgens oestrogens testosterone	gonads & genitalia 2° sexual characteristics	supports & maintains the sexual organs & characteristics of the body
Adrenal Medulla	CATECHOLAMINES adrenaline, noradrenaline, dopamine	Brain / BVs, Heart Liver Whole Body	Fight/Flight Responses ↑ B[glucose] constricts BVs ↑ BP redirects BF to the SKM
Hypothalamus	RELEASING FACTORS CRF / GRF/ GnRF / PRF / TRF	Ant. Pit.	Causes release of trophic Hs
	INHIBITING FACTORS GIF / PIF / SRIF		Stops the release of trophic Hs
	DOPAMINE	Brain	↑ movement Produces *good feelings*
	RELEASING FACTORS	Post Pit.	releases/transports factors which retain water & release milk
Ovaries	ACTIVIN	Ant. Pit.	↑ FSH
	INHIBIN (granulosa cells)		↓ FSH

Ovaries (cont.)	OESTROGENS	Whole Body Uterus	↑ development differentiation growth & maintenance of the ♀ genitalia & gonad & 2° sexual characteristics
	PROGESTERONE	Uterus	maintenance of the pregnancy
	TESTOSTERONE ~1/7 of ♂		↑ libido
Pancreas α cells	GCG	Liver	↑ B[glucose]
β cells	INS	Whole Body	↓ B[glucose] ↑ fat & protein metabolism
γ cells	SOMATOSTATIN	Ant. Pit.	↓ Trophic Hs
	PaP	Pancreas	feedback loop to suppress pancreatic secretions
Parathyroid Glands	PTH	Bone	↑ B[Ca] ↑ bone resorption ↓ B[PO4]
Pineal Gland	MELATONIN	Whole Body	controls circadian rhythms
Pituitary Anterior	TROPHIC Hs ACTH / GH / LPH / PRL	Adrenal cortex Whole body Mammary glands	↑ steroid Hs & grth of adrenal cortex ↑ growth & differentiation ↑ protein production. (inc. milk) ↑ ANABOLIC processes
	STIMULATING Hs FSH / LH / MSH / TSH	Ovary / Testes / Hair & Skin / Thyroid	↑ follicles & CL ↑ spermatogenesis & interstitial cells ↑ libido & appetite ↑ pigmentation ↑ THs
Pituitary Posterior	Oxytocin ADH	Uterus Kidney	Hs released or transported through here from the hypothalamus - to lactate / instigate childbirth / retain water / increase thirst

Placenta	hCG	Ovary	promote & maintain CL in pregnancy
		Immune System	Inhibit IR towards embryo;
	CRF	Uterus	Determines length of gestation & timing of childbirth sudden ↑ B[ ] at birth.
	HPL INHIBIN RELAXIN OESTROGENS PROGESTINS		↑ Insulin & IGF-1 production ↓ FSH Similar to ovarian follicle oestrogen Supports pregnancy
Prostate gland	DHT		↑ prostate size
Testes	OESTROGENS	Testes, Prostate	maintenance of the ♂ germ cells
	ANDROSTENEDIONE		acts as an oestrogen
	TESTOSTERONES	Testes Whole Body	↑ development differentiation growth & maintenance of the ♂ genitalia & gonad & 2° sexual characteristics ↑ Spermatogenesis ↑ SKM ↑ cartilage grth - voice changes
Testes *(cont.)*	DHT *A metabolite of TESTOSTERONE but more potent*	♂ 2° sexual characteristics	Essential role in formation of ♂ embryo 's external genitals, ↑ prostate ↑ HFs on the body ↑ baldness on the head dev. diff. growth & maintenance of the male sex organs, 2° sexual characteristics
Thymus	THYMOSIN	immune system	↑ differentiation WBCs-formation of T cells maintains supports ↑ WBCs

| Thyroid | T3 / T4 | Whole Body | ↑ cellular metabolism
↑ BMR
↑ ????
(↑ in pregancy) |
| | CALCITONIN
CGRP | Bone | ↑ osteoblasts/bone construction;
↓ B[Ca2+] |

Examples of non-Endocrine Organs that secrete Hs/ H-like substances

Organ	Secretions
Bone	BONE MORPHOGENETIC PROTEIN (BMP), OSTEOCALCIN
Brain	DOPAMINE (BNP)
Heart	NATRIURETIC PEPTIDES (ANP, BNP)
Intestines	CCK, GIP, SECRETIN, MOTILIN, VIP, ENTEROGLUCAGON, ENTEROSTATIN
Liver/other	ANGIOTENSIN II, INSULIN-LIKE GROWTH FACTORS (IGF-1, IGF-2)
Kidneys	ANGIOTENSIN, RENIN, ERYTHROPOIETIN (EPO), CALCITRIOL, PROSTAGLANDINS (PGs)
Salivary Gland	EPIDERMAL GROWTH FACTOR (EGF)
Skeletal Muscle	IRISIN
Stomach	GASTRIN, GHRELIN, HISTAMINE, SUBSTANCE P

Adipose Tissue - Changes in Obesity

Schema
A normal adipose cells
B dysfunctional adipose cells obesity changes

AT changes in the obese individual & becomes sensitized. The tissue is in a constant pro-If state, insulin resistive and hypoxic. New BVs form, the ECM is modified & the fat cells swell, as they take on more lipid, & secrete more FAs. The lipid vacuole is not as protected as the perilipin - covering protective protein layer, is thinner allowing more TGAs to be exposed to lipases, in the cytosol. This places the body in a sensitive state more prone to chronic If, cardiovascular disease & developing DM2. It also is a more conducive environment for the development of cancerous change.

		changes in obesity (0)
1	collagen / proteoglycans	additional fibres & matrix laid down
2	capillaries	+++ vascularity
3	adipocyte	++++ in size ± numbers ↓ in insulin binding proteins ↑IR
4	macrophage	activated / actively secreting cytokines + other if factors pro-If
5	fibrotic deposits	increased amounts laid down
6	laminin	additional deposits laid down
7	fibronectin	additional deposits laid down
	lipids / FFAs	increased amounts released into the circulation
	Leptin	increased secretion, which affect appetite & hunger levels in the hypothalamus

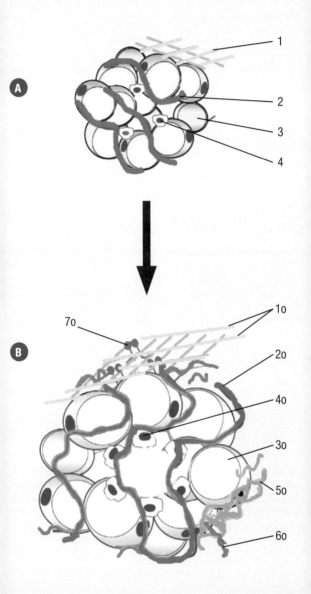

Adipose Tissue (AT)

Roles in Endocrinology

AT passively stores excess carbon in the form of FAs & TGAs. It is the primary storage site of E in the body. It plays a major role in thermogenesis, insulation & protection of its enclosed Ts & organs.

AT is highly innervated with noradrenergic fibres, & contains: endothelial cells, fibrocytes, mØ, stem cells & WBCs.

AT synthesizes & secretes numerous substances involved in E homeostasis & the IfR. Most of these substances are **pro-If AKA adipocytokines AKA adipokines**, which leads to its involvement in the development of: atherosclerosis, hypertension & IR.

AT is a factor in: angiogenesis, appetite regulation, fertility and glucose & lipid metabolism.

Brown adipose tissue (1) (BAT) makes up a small % of AT. It is found mainly around the aorta & vital organs, & involved in thermogenesis (heat production). The adipocytes are smaller with multiple lipid droplets. They have large numbers of mitochondria & cytochromes

White adipose tissue (2) (WAT) is the main form of AT. It is composed of large rounded cells (adipocytes) with > 90% taken up by a single fat droplet in a loose highly vascularised CT. WAT is concentrated around organs of the thorax (visceral fat) & subcutaneously (sc fat).

Regulation of Lipid Metabolism in Adipocytes

FFAs are released from AT via hydrolysis of TGAs via **H-sensitive lipase (HSL)**.

FFAs then circulate & are taken up by cells for their E needs, see Lipoproteins .

Catecholamines & glucagon bind to adipocytes triggering activation of **adenylate cyclase** which ↑ cAMP. cAMP activates PKA which activates HSL via phosphorylation.

Feeding ↓ TGA lipolysis via Insulin.

Insulin activates **protein phosphatase-1** which deactivates **HSL** via dephosphorylation.

AMPK also deactivates **HSL**, & ensures that the FFAs released into the BS are not in excess to the body's needs.

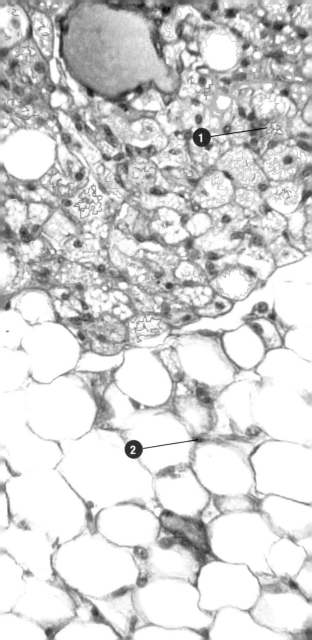

AT & the Inflammatory Response (IfR)

Obesity causes ↑ AT released cytokines, putting the individual in a pro-If state, & promoting the development of IR & DM2, it also ↑ Leptin which further stimulates AT mass ↑, by stimulating the appetite and suppressing satiety, so forming a positive feedback loop.

In particular levels of ILs, MCP & resident mØs are increased, in the obese, but Adiponectin which is anti-inflammatory is suppressed.

Visceral WAT secretes a higher percentage of the circulating IL-6 than sc WAT, hence central obesity is considered a higher disease risk than sc fat.

TNF directly inhibits insulin receptors by phosphorylation leading to ↑ IR as well as inhibiting Adiponectin, which is anti-inflammatory.

TNF also ↓ endo nitric oxide synthase (eNOS) resulting in ↓ levels of NO. This leads ↑ oxidative stress & accumulation of ROS, causing transcriptional changes & synthesis of more cytokines, & ↑ If processes. Lymphocytes (T-cells & B-cells) are physically associated w/n the LNs to AT which surrounds the LNs & allows for 2-way paracrine interactions b/n the lymph & AT.

Cytokines & Hs of Adipocytes

AT produces & releases a vast array of protein signals, which vary depending upon its anatomical region. Visceral WAT is involved in the development of: IR, DM2 & cardiovascular disease, whereas sc WAT is not, & the substances they produce or express as receptors reflect this.

Factors released from WAT include :

Acute Inflammatory phase proteins -e.g. CRP, SAA
Adhesion molecules e.g. ICAM, VCAM,
Angiogenic growth factors e.g. angiopoietin, VEGF
Chemokines e.g. MCP, MIP
Compliment-like factors e.g. adiponectin, adipsin, ASP

Cytokines: e.g. ILs, MIP, TNF
Extracellular components e.g. collagen, fibronectin, **MMP**
Growth factors e.g. FGF, HGF, IGF, NGF, TGF, VEGF,
Metabolic process factors e.g. adipocyte-FA-binding protein, Leptin
Other e.g. COX pathway products, PG, renin - angiotensin system

Membrane Receptors synthesised by AT include receptors for:

Adiponectin
Angiotensin II
Gastrin

Glucagon
GH
Insulin

Nuclear Receptors synthesised by AT include receptors for:

Androgens
Glucocorticoids
Oestrogens
Progesterones

THs
Vitamin D
Peroxisome proliferator

Adiponectin, Leptin & Resistin major Hs of AT

H secreted by AT (& other major sources)	ratios	Tissues affected	stimulated by	inhibited by	Major Action
ADIPONECTIN AKA adipocyte complement factor 1q-related protein (ACRP30) AKA AdipoQ (adipocytes) protein H	♀ > ♂ thin > fat normal > DM type II	SKM > Liver > Brain	insulin "thinness"	adrenergic stimulation catecholamines glucocorticoids TNF obesity	↑ insulin sensitivity ↑ FA oxidation ↓ TNF *(endo cells & SM prolif in BVs)* ↓ glucose release from Ts (liver)
LEPTIN (adipocytes, mammary glds, intestine, mu, placenta) protein H	fat > thin levels directly correlate with body fat levels ♀ > ♂	arcuate nuc of hypothalamus - *appetite centre* - ↑ appetite suppression m∅ - ↑ If - pro-inflammatory BVs - endothelium ↑ atherosclerosis thymus - ↑ T cells	AT, oestrogens sex steroids, glucocorticoids, cytokines & toxins released during acute If (not in chronic If)	catecholamines Sym Ns	regulates of overall body wgt by limiting food intake & ↑ E expenditure. ↑ IF responses, BP, & bone mass pre-disposing a person to AI
RESISTIN AKA FIZZ3 (m∅, adipocytes, spleen, monocytes, lung, kidney, bone marrow, placenta) protein H		AT - ↑ adipocyte differentiation liver ↑ hepatic glucose production & glucose intolerance BVs SM & endo cells ↑ IfR, ↑ adhesion molecs			pro-If - in If zone ↑ IR in the liver

Breast development

Schema of breast glands & nipple
A   hormonal control of glandular development
B   anatomy of breast alveolus
C   anatomy of the breast nipple

The immature breast (i) breast begins to mature at puberty (1) developing ducts & glandular T under H influence (ii), along with an increase in AT. This matures (2) & further development (iii) only occurs with pregnancy (3), when the T begins to lactate (iv). The breast T remains constant until menopause when it is no longer supported by oestrogen. The glands regress & AT ↓ causing the skin to pucker. Drooping occurs due to changes in the supportive collagen fibres.

1   **Oestrogen, GH, Adrenal steroids influence the initial changes in the breast T,**
      promoting ductal growth
2   **Oestrogen, Progesterone, PRL, GH & Adrenal steroids cause maturation of the breast T**
      forming lobules and alveolar development
3   **PRL, Oxytocin promote the synthesis & secretion of milk for lactation**
4   **myoepithelial cells - contractile cells**
5   **alveolar cells lining the ducts**
6   **lumen of the alveoli containing milk when lactating**
7   **collecting duct**
8   **BS - arteriole & venule**
9   **capillaries**
10 **mammary duct**
11 **lactiferous duct**
12 **areola**
13 **nipple**

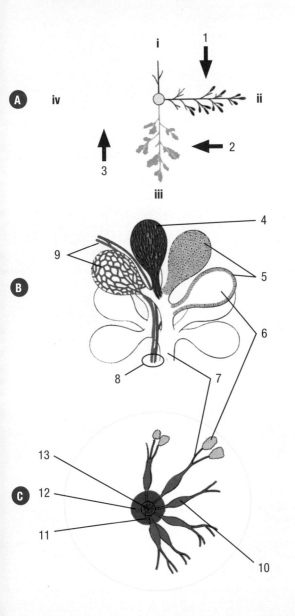

Hypothalamus

Schema of basal nuclei AKA basal ganglia of the hypothalamus

The hypothalamus consists of a number of GM nuclei AKA Basal nuclei AKA Basal ganglia centred & named around the 3rd ventricle (V). These nuclei interconnect with the CC via the thalamus & coordinate a number of bodily functions via Hs neuropeptides & neural connections.

1   post. hypothalamic nucleus

2   dorso-medial nucleus

3   venromedial nucleus

4   pre-mammillary nucleus

5   medial mammillary nucleus

6   lateral mammillary nucleus

7   mammillary body

8   post. pit.

9   ant. pit.

10   portal hypophyseal vessels

11   sup. hypophyseal art.

12   medial eminence

13   optic chiasm

14   arcuate nucleus

15   suprachiasmatic nucleus

16   supra-optic nucleus

17   pre-optic area

18   ant. hypothalamic area

19   paraventricular nucleus

20   dorsal hypothalamic nucleus

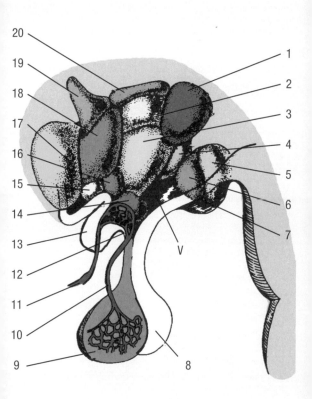

Hypothalamic control of Appetite

Schema of Hormonal feedback to the Hypothalamus involved in hunger & satiety

The hypothalamus is composed of several nuclei, 5 of which are involved in feeding & satiety:

the arcuate nucleus of the hypothalamus (ARC),

the dorsomedial hypothalamic nucleus (DMN), &

the ventromedial hypothalamic nucleus (VMN) all located in the tuberal medial area.

The ARC is involved in control of feeding behaviour as well as secretion of various RFs for pituitary Hs;

the DMN is involved in stimulating GIT activity, & the VMN is involved in satiety.

The lateral hypothalamic nuclei are responsible for **hunger**, while the medial hypothalamic nuclei are responsible for the sensations of **satiety**.

Appetite is complex resulting from the integration of the multiple signals to the hypothalamus, which are: **neural signals**, from the CC, & cranial Ns

H signals e.g. INS (pancreas), Leptin (AT), PYY (SI) & Ghrelin (stomach) and

nutrient signals e.g. glucose, FFAs & AAs.

The H signals bind to receptors on orexigenic &/or anorexigenic Ns in the ARC of the hypothalamus, which release either the orexigenic neuropeptides NPY & AgRP or the anorexigenic neuropeptides CART & the POMC-derived peptide α-MSH.

These neuropeptides travel along axons to 2° Ns in the paraventricular nucleus (PVN).

The ultimate effects of these signalling cascades are changes in the sensation of hunger & satiety in the NTS.

1   **PYY from the SI**
2   **INS from the pancreas**
3   **Leptin from AT**
4   **Ghrelin from the stomach**
5   **orexigenic Ns (Hunger Inducing Ns) containing :**
        neuropeptide tyrosine = NPY
        agouti-related peptide (antagonizes α-MSH) = AgRP
6   **anorexigenic Ns (satiation inducing Ns) containing :**
        cocaine & amphetamine-regulated transcript = CART
        pro-opiomelanocoticotropin = POMC
7   **2nd order Ns**
8   **nucleus of the solitary tract (NTS) satiety centre in the hypothalamus**
9   **3rd Ventricle of the brain**
10 **Arcuate nucleus -**
11 **Paraventricular nucleus**

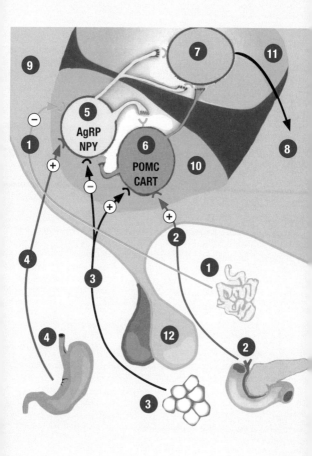

Hypothalamus Overview

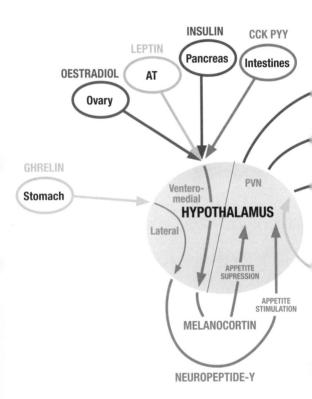

© A. L. Neill

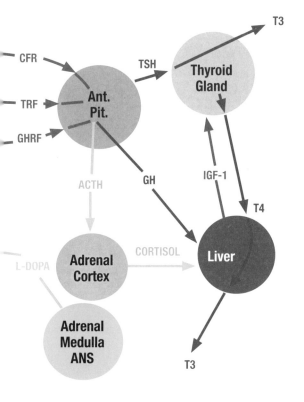

Kidney – functioning unit
Nephron

Schema of the nephron & the passage of fluids in the tubules
A = Cortex B = Medulla (inner & outer medulla)

The kidney's primary function is the selected filtration of the blood fluid contents. The main functioning unit for this is the nephron. B is passed at a high P through a knot of capillaries (3) & the filtered fluid collected in the surrounding capsule. The fluid almost completely devoid of plasma proteins & passes through a series of tubules (4,5,6) which depending upon the fluid balance of the body will concentrate or dilute this solution, through a series of active transport system under H influence. At the level of the CDs the final composition of the urine is determined & passes into the renal pelvis forming the urine.

1 **afferent arteriole entering the glomerulus**
2 **efferent arteriole leaving the glomerulus**
3 **glomerulus - capillaries - w/n the capsule**
   c = cortical glomerulus - shorter LoH stopping in the outer medulla
   j = juxta medullary glomerulus longer LoH into the inner medulla-
4 **PCT -closest to the glomerulus - in the renal cortex, site of AA, GLUCOSE & Na conservation. Aquaporins (AKA water channels) also allow water to leave the tubules, influenced by DOPAMINE.**
5 **loop tubules = Loop of Henle (LoH) thick & thin segments - thin segments allow water to passively leave the tubules under osmotic P. The longer the LoH the greater the capacity to concentrate the urine.**
6 **DCT - cells of this tubule & the thick ascending LoH make up the MD.**
7 **macula densa (MD)- part of the JGA. This is the site of EPO synthesis.**
8 **CD collect fluid from several DCTs and travel into the renal pelvis & through the concentrated gradient of the medulla. Depending upon the fluid balance in the body, may move out of the DCs under AHD & ALDOSTERONE influence. Both Hs conserve water allowing it to leave via the aquaporins to leave the CDs.**
9 **papillary tubules**
10 **arcuate arteries**
11 **renal pelvis**

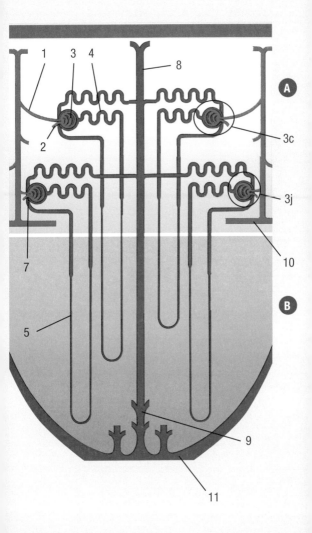

Pancreas

A Macroscopic - Anterior cutaway showing pancreatic duct
B Schema of exocrine & endocrine functions

The pancreas is a grey comma-shaped organ up to 15cm long,
fixed to the posterior abdominal wall - lying in the upper abdomen
and extending from the R – where its head inserts into the "C" of the
duodenum – to the L where its tail extends into the hilum of
the spleen.

The pancreas has small endocrine islets – islets of Langerhan's –
sitting amidst serous exocrine glands which secrete digestive enzymes
into the second part of the duodenum (descending duodenum). So it
demonstrates the 2 forms of BS to these different gland types. The
islets contain at least 4 different types of cells but the main cells types
are the glucagon producing α cells (10-20%), which liberate glucose
from the cells and the insulin producing β cells (60-80%), which
allow entrance of sugars into the cells for use & storage. Somatostatin
secreted by the δ cells regulate the use of sugar by affecting the α
& β cells directly. The serous glands secrete enzymes in an alkaline
solution to both digest the chyme from the stomach and to neutralize
its acidity.

1   **interlobular collecting duct**
2   **serous gland**
3   **acinar cell of the serous gland = exocrine gland**
4   **pancreatic islet = endocrine gland**
   a = alpha cells
   b = beta cells
   v = capillaries b/n the islet cell
5   **CT stroma = septum b/n the glands**
6   **intercalated ducts**
7   **a & v with capillaries traversing through the islets**

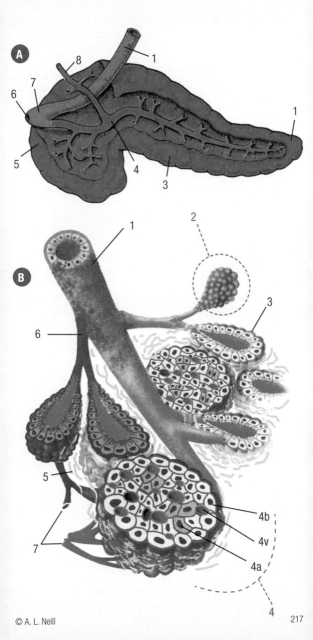

Parathyroid & Thyroid glands *in situ*

Macroscopic - cellular schema –

A in the neck- across the trachea flanked by the carotid arteries

B parathyroid gland embedded in the thyroid gland

C thyroid follicles

D parathyroid cellular arrangement

The pancreas is a grey comma-shaped organ up to 15cm long, fixed to the posterior abdominal wall - lying in the upper abdomen and extending from the R – where its head inserts into the "C" of the duodenum – to the L where its tail extends into the hilum of the spleen.

The parathyroid glands are 4 (range 3-6) small beanlike mustard coloured endocrine glands which are embedded in the back of the thyroid gland, either side of the trachea. They are not visible nor palpable on examination & separated from the thyroid only by a thin shared capsule. Hence the name- "near" the thyroid). The normal size for each gland is b/n 30-200mg 2X4X6mm, ($\female > \male$), but there is considerable variation. Adenomas grow up to 500mg. They act independently of the thyroid.

Parathyroid glands are responsible for the Calcium (Ca) & Phosphate (P) levels in the body via the Parathyroid hormone (PTH). PTH works on a feedback loop stimulating Ca mobilization in response to ↓ B[Ca]. Constant high levels of PTH will result in bone loss & OP.

1 **thyroid**

2 **parathyroid**

3 **follicle colloid**

4 **CT stroma of the glds**

5 **follicular cells of the thyroid - single epithelial layer**

6 **parafollicular cells of the thyroid**

7 **capsule**

8 **chief cells -produce & release PTH**

9 **oxyphil cells -function ?**

10 **BVs**

11 **trachea**

© A. L. Neill

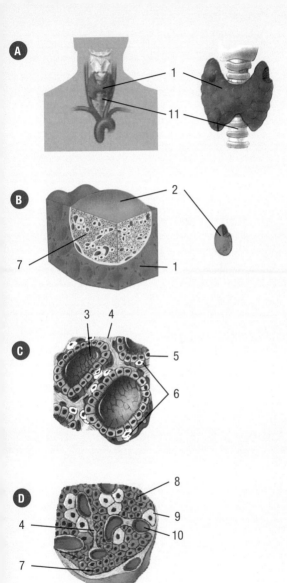

Parathyroid & Thyroid - Blood Supply

Arterial supply

Lateral view with cartilage wall removed to show inside

Medial view - cartilage wall removed

The BS of the larynx, parathyroid and thyroid are related intimately
Hence voice changes may be a sign of pathologies in these areas.

1 **carotid arteries c = common / e = external /
   i = internal**
2 **lingual arteries**
3 **hyoid arteries i = infrahyoid / s = suprahyoid a**
4 **laryngeal i = inferior / s = superior**
5 **thyroid art i = inferior / s = superior**
6 **cricothyroid m**
7 **thyrocervical trunk**
8 **subclavian a**
9 **aorta**
10 **Hyoid bone**
11 **cricoid cartilage**
12 **epiglottis**
13 **thyroid**
14 **trachea**

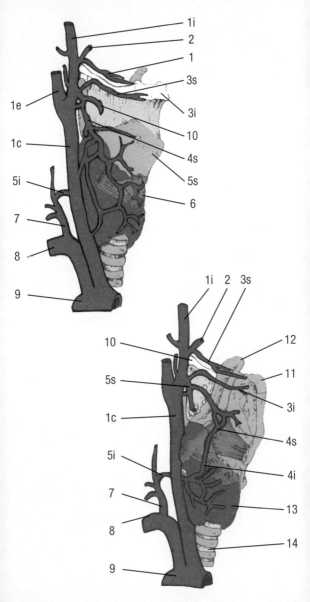

1i

2

1

3s

3i

10

1e

4s

1c

5s

5i

6

7

8

9

1i 2 3s

10

12

11

5s

3i

1c

4s

5i

4i

7

13

8

14

9

© A. L. Neill

Pineal gland AKA Epiphysis Cerebri AKA The Third eye

Macroscopic view
Sagittal section through part of the brain

The pineal gland is a pine cone shaped gland of diencephalon (6X6 mm). It has a strong BS considering its small size, and acts as a bridge b/n the nervous & endocrine systems similar to the Hypothalamus / Pituitary glands, converting sensory input of the SymNS to H signals. The main H produced is Melatonin. The pineal gland influences: sexual development, the onset of menarche & menopause, male puberty & the body's circadian rhythm (sleep wake cycle). It is photosensitive, despite being in the centre of the brain. It often calcifies with age, & accumulates fluoride selectively. The effect on its function in these circumstances is not known.

1   corpus callosum
2   choroid plexus of 3rd ventricle
3   intermediate mass of the thalamus
4   commissure
    a = anterior
    p = posterior
5   optic chiasm
6   hypothalamus
7   pituitary gland
8   mammillary body
9   pons
10 cerebral aqueduct
11 cerebellum
12 superior cervical sympathetic ganglia
13 sympathetic input to the pineal gland
14 pineal gland

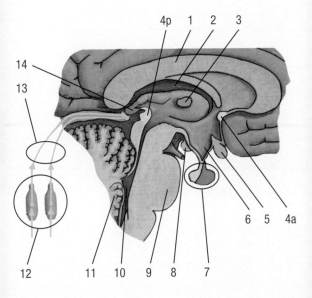

Pituitary AKA Hypophysis
Anterior & Posterior

Pituitary In Situ - inferior, sagittal, in the sella turcica, in the cavernous sinus
Pituitary anterior & posterior relationship with the hypothalamus

The pituitary gland is really 2 glands - originating from 2 different sources. The more adenoidal is the anterior lobe which releases a large number of Hs controlled by the RF or IF of the hypothalamus. The posterior lobe is connected to the hypothalamus by the infundibulum which carries the Ns from the hypothalamus. These Ns are intimately related to the pituicytes, specialized cells which engulf the axons & release the 2 Hs of this lobe.

1. **hypothalamus**
   p= paraventricular nucleus / s = supraoptic nucleus
2. **axons**
3. **hypothalamic Ns - secrete CRF GRF + GIF, GnRF, PIF, TRF**
   stimulating & inhibiting factors of the Hs of the ant pituitary
4. **optic chiasm**
5. **superior hypophyseal a**
6. **hypophyseal capillary plexi**
   p = primary / s = secondary
7. **hypophyseal portal v**
   6 + 7 = hypophyseal / pituitary portal system
8. **Hs of the ant pituitary - ACTH, FSH, GH. LH, PRL, TSH**
9. **infundibulum AKA pituitary stalk**
10. **hypothalmic -hypophyseal N tract**
11. **inf hypophyseal AKA inf. pituitary a**
12. **Hs of the post pituitary ADH AKA Vasopressin, Oxytocin**
13. **axon terminals - travel into the post. lobe**

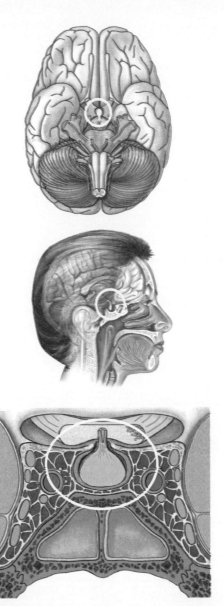

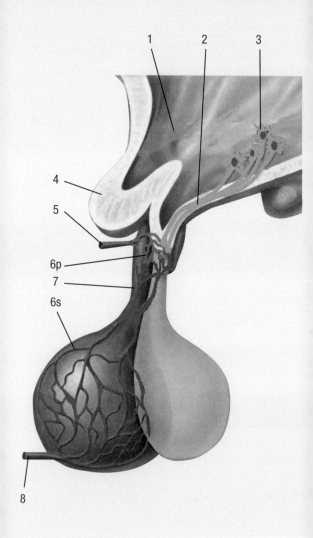

© A. L. Neill

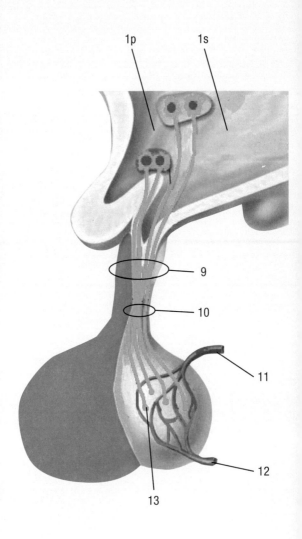

Pituitary gland

Schema overview

1 **hypothalamus - neurons interact with the cells &/or BVs of the pituitary gld directly to affect its secretions**

2 **primary capillary plexus**

3 **optic chiasm**

4 **pituitary portal system**

5 **pituitary gland**
   a = ant. pituitary AKA adenohypophysis
   p = post. pituitary AKA neurohypophysis

6 **basophilic cells secrete**
   a = ACTH - stimulates the adrenal gld
   b = TSH - stimulates the thyroid
   c = FSH - stimulates maturation of ovary follicles & oestrogen secretion
   c = FSH - stimulates spermatogenesis
   d = LH - stimulates ovulation
   d = LH - stimulates testosterone secretion

7 **acidophilic cells secrete**
   a = prolactin - stimulates milk secretion
   b = GH - causes hyperglycaemia
       - elevates free fatty acids
       - stimulates bone growth

8 **neurohypophyseal cells secrete**
   a = oxytocin - causes uterine contractions & milk ejection
   b = ADH - causes water retention

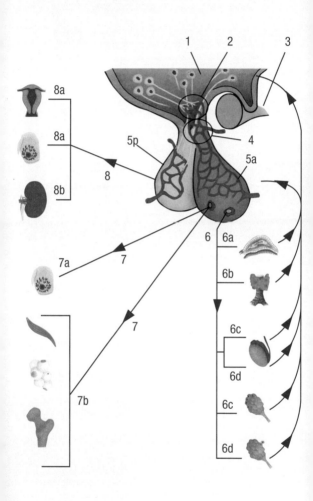

Pituitary - anterior AKA Adenohypophysis AKA Pars Distalis
Trophic releasing cells AKA Tropic cells

Schema of relationship b/n hypothalamus (A) portal circulation (B) & trophic cells (C)

The anterior pituitary gland is an extension of the palate. The 3 types of cells present resemble glandular cells which react to the RFs of the hypothalamus, carried down to them via the portal system. The BV become sinusoids when they reach the ant. pit, allowing the direct entry and exit of RFs & Hs into the BS.

1   **capillary in the brain - note BBB tight Junction b/n endothelial cells - astrocyte & BM layers**

2   **synapses b/n Ns from higher centres and hypothalamic Ns**

3   **secretory granules RFs & IFs + synaptic vesicles of neurotransmitters - (note these are PPs or proteins)**

4   **vesicles in the axon of the hypothalamic cell (10,000 axonal processes may course through here)**

5   **capillaries of the median eminence - BBB - beginning of the portal vessels**

6   **"secretions" of the hypothalamic Ns carried down to the ant. pit. - these are RFs & IFs which will stimulate or inhibit the pit. Hs**

7   **astrocyte - processes may be present at the level of the portal vessels**

8   **portal BVs b/n the primary and secondary capillary plexi -no BBB present at this point**

9   **BM- sometimes the only barrier b/n the lumen of the barrier and the cm of the trophic cells of the ant. pit.**

10 **sinusoidal capillary with gaps in the endothelial barrier -**

11 **Trophic cells of the ant pit - 3 main types - characterized by their staining affinities with H&E**
    a = acidophils (somatotrophs & lactotrophs)
    b = basophils (thyrotrophs, gonadotrophs & corticotrophs)
    c = chromophobes which are either depleted cells w/o H granules or stem cells

12 **secretory granules of the trophic cells**

13 **substances present in the BV lumen are**
    RFs & IFs of the hypothalamus + secretions from the ant. pit.

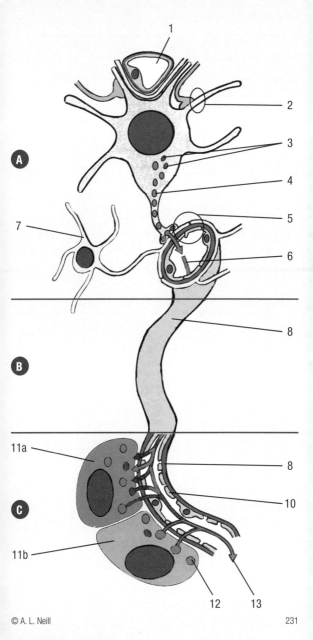

A

B

C

1

2

3

4

5

6

7

8

8

10

11a

11b

12

13

© A. L. Neill

Pituitary - posterior AKA Neurohypophysis AKA Pars Nervosa
Pituicyte

LP - Schema of relationship b/n pituicyte & axon from the hypothalamus
HP - Cell structure pituicytes & axons

The posterior pituitary gland is an extension of the hypothalamus. It contains large irregular cells called pituicytes which closely associate with the hypothalamic Ns & bind to the capillaries. Their foot processes retract to allow direct contact with the axon & its H secretions, OXYTOCIN & VASOPRESSIN. Herring bodies (HBs) AKA neurosecretory vesicles of Hs & their carrier molecules, as well as many other vesicles are found throughout the axon length forming dilatations along its length. Most vesicles are found at the axon terminus.

1   **axon from the hypothalamus**
2   **Herring bodies**
        other secretory granules (2g) & synaptic vesicles (2v)
3   **microfilaments - in axons and pituicytes**
4   **pituicyte - only in the post. pituitary**
5   **capillary -**
        f= fenestrated region allows for the passage of large molecules
6   **axon terminus**
7   **pericapillary space opened via pituicyte pseudopod retraction - allow free passage of secretions**
8   **mitochondria**

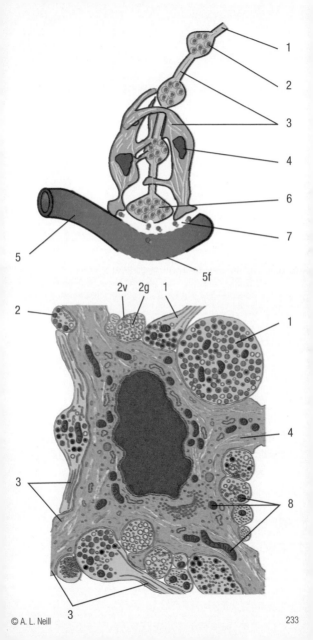

Placenta

Schema of villous formation & BF b/n mother & foetus

The Placenta is an organ used to allow nutrients to be delivered to the growing embryo from the mother w/o mixing of the 2 bloods. Blood flows from the mother through the placental septa and the spiral arteries and bathes the stems filles with embryonic BVs, before draining away through the endometrial veins.

It acts like a giant CL - producing Hs to support the pregnancy and taking over the CL role.

Trophoblasts from the placenta and foetus support the mucosa of the uterine wall, suppress the IR of the mother, and allow many of the maternal Hs to pass through to support the foetal development and differentiation.

1. myometrium
2. decidua basalis
3. endometrial spiral a - shooting maternal blood into the intervillous spaces through a complex capillary system
4. placental septa
5. cotyledons
6. endometrial v - drains the blood from the cotyledons after it has bathed the embryonic villi
7. amnion
8. chlorionic plate
9. main stem villus - covered with embryonic tissue
10. umbilical a & v (2 veins)
11. villus containing convoluted a & v from the embryo
12. villus stump

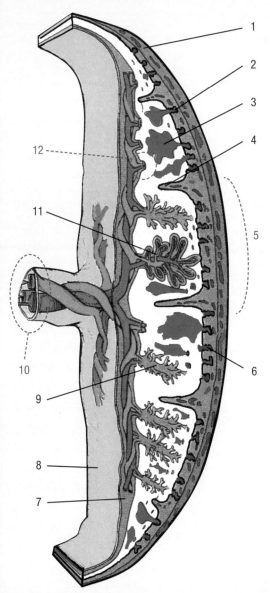

Prostate & Seminal Vesicles (SV)

A schema of seminal vesicles & prostate posterior view
B transverse section of prostate

The SVs are composed of tubular alveoli & the mucosa is thrown into an intricate system of folds with the epithelium overlaying the LP. SVs overlie the prostate gland & join the ampulla of the deferens to form the beginning of ejaculatory ducts. Secretion of the SVs constitutes the main (50%) & the last fraction of the ejaculate. It coagulates the dispersed liquid ejaculate (with semenogelin I, a protein specific to the SV) & ↑ sperm motility. Prostatic secretions supply peptides which feed the released sperm. The sex differentiation, growth & maintenance of SVs & the prostate gland are dependent upon Androgens. Endogenous ↑ B[testosterone] ↑ the secretory activity of the SVs, & prostate. SV & prostate secretions are also important for: stability of sperm chromatin & suppression of the immune activity in the ♀ reproductive tract, to avoid rejection of spermatozoa & embryo (in case of fertilization) that have foreign Ags. The function of the prostate & the SVs are essential for fertility.

SVs possess **5-α-reductase**, which converts Testosterone to DHT, the active H, & receptors for LH & hCG, which also stimulate spermatogenesis, via Testosterone. The SVs & prostate share the same BS, & hormonal influences. Products of the SVs which ↑ sperm motility are: K+, HCO3 & Mg & Prolactin. SVs secrete Ags which prevent ♀ IR against spermatozoa & embryo, & ↓ the effects of maternal WBC on the spermatozoa. Zn bound to metallothionein, is secreted by the Prostate & stabilizes the sperm chromatin at the correct levels regulated by the SVs. INS is also secreted by the SVs although is function is unclear.

1 1 **ductus deferens**
      a = ampulla
2 **SV**
3 **urethra**
      c = crest
      p = prostatic
4 **parenchyma of the prostate**
5 **prostatic utricle**
6 **ejaculatory duct**
7 **capsule**

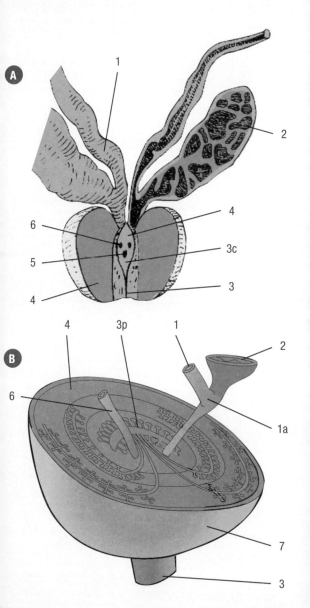

Testes

Macroscopic view
Sagittal section showing interior & BS
Schema of tubules to show continuity from the testis

The testes are the site of spermatogenesis. The sperm once matured breakaway from the epithelial lining of the seminiferous tubules from which they are derived & proceed to the epididymis, & then through to the VD to the seminal vesicles.

1   vas deferens
2   epididymis
      d = ductus epididyis
3   vasa efferentes
4   vas aberans
5   tunica albuginea
6   fibrous septum
7   lobule
8   rete testis in the mediastinum of the testis
9   pampiniform plexus
10   internal spermatic artery
11   seminiferous tubules

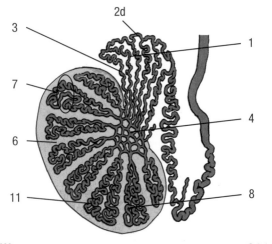

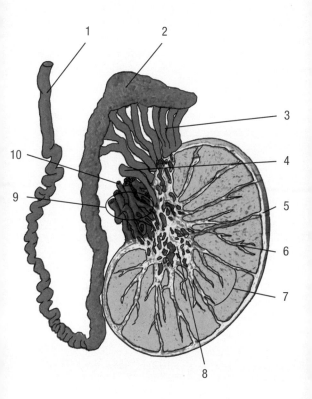

Thyroid & Parathyroid glands

Macroscopic view–
Anterior
Posterior

The thyroid gland is a butterfly shaped encapsulated organ which straddles the trachea at T1. It has 2 lobes & a connecting isthmus. It may occasionally have an additional pyramidal lobe, which lies along & up the trachea. The normal weight is b/n 15-20g. It is derived from the invagination of the pharyngeal epithelium & descends from the anterior of the neck.

The post. surface encloses the 4 parathyroid glands in separate capsules.

Their functions are not related.

1 **thyroid cartilage**
2 **cricoid cartilage - site of the pyramidal lobe if present**
3 **isthmus**
4 **inferior parathyroid gland + lower pole of the thyroid**
5 **body of thyroid - lobe**
6 **upper pole of the thyroid**
7 **inferior constrictor of the pharynx**
8 **post surface of the thyroid**
9 **superior parathyroid gland**
10 **oesophagus**
11 **transition b/n pharynx and oesophagus - Killen's triangle**

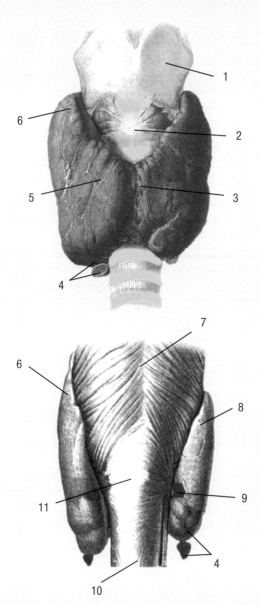

© A. L. Neill

Thyroid gland - cellular changes

Schema

A *Synthesizing cell*

B *Resting cell*

C *Secreting cell*

The thyroid gland synthesizes, stores & releases thyroid Hs (T3 & T4), and these activities may all be occurring at once w/in the thyroid gland. Although an endocrine gland the H secretion is stored outside the cell as a colloid, and must be retrieved, via pseudopodal resorption, transported across the cell & modified before release.

1 **AAs in the BV - absorbed into the cell**

2 **go to rER for synthesis of thyroglobulin + peroxidase**

3 **go to Golgi for added sugars**

4 **release of thyroglobulin + peroxidase into the follicle**

5 **iodide absorbed from the BS**

6 **released and converted to iodine by peroxidase in the follicle**

7 **formation of the thyroid Hs T3 & T4 - which then combine with the colloid**

8 **colloid storage material**

9 **mv - range in size depending upon the state of the cell - longer when active**

10 **Junctional complexes b/n cells - to prevent passage of material**

11 **large numbers of mitos when cell is active**

12 **pseudopod - to phagocytose large colloid droplets**

13 **combination colloid + H**

14 **lysosome - which combines with phagosome & liberates the Hs - T3 & T4**

15 **release of Hs directly into the BV**

16 **BM - of gland and BVs**

17 **capillary lumen**

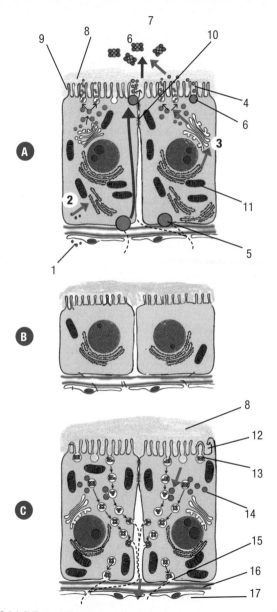

Thyroid gland - H production

Schema of the 3 different metabolic states of the follicular cells

1   AAs in the BV - move into the cell
2   go to rER for synthesis of thyroglobulin + peroxidase
3   go to Golgi for added sugars
4   thyroglobulin + peroxidase in vacuoles - note mv ~.2μm
5   released into the follicle
6   iodide absorbed from the BS
7   released & converted to iodine by peroxidase in the follicle - note active darkened nucleus
8   columnar cell - reduced to cuboidal
9   mv shortened, flatter, separated from colloid
10 colloid storage material
11 resting nucleus, reduced organelles including mitochondria (not shown)
12 pseudopodial extension growing from the elongated mv - up to 1.2μm
13 movement to engulf colloid
14 vesicle of colloid ic AKA phagosome
15 fusion of lysosome with phagosome
16 proteolytic enzymes breakdown the thyroglobulin
17 formation of the thyroid H T4 - released 10X more than T3
18 formation of the thyroid H T3 -- small amounts main source is the conversion from T4 in the liver
19 Hs released into the BS via capillaries - fenestrated endothelium

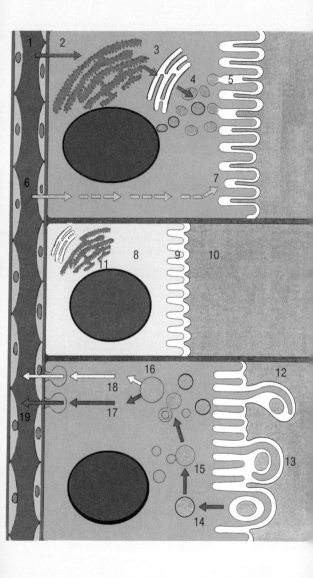

Hyper & Hypo Thyroidism

	HYPERTHYROIDISM	FEATURES	HYPOTHYROIDISM
	+ / -	birth defects / developmental problems	+++ / +++
	↑↑↑	BMR / E consumption	↓↓↓
	↑↑ running thoughts / distraction anxiety hyper-reflexia / ↑↑	CNS CHANGES appetite mental activity / ability moods reflexes / reactivity	↓ memory loss / fogging depression / mood swings hyporeflexia / ↓
	↑ IR / ↑ B[glucose] / ↑ DM1&2	DM	associated with DM2 ↑
1	thin, fine	eyebrows	loss of lateral 1/3
2	exophthalmia (protrusion) strabismus / staring gaze	eyes / look	↑ ocular P / dull non focused gaze floaters ++
3	proptosis (retraction) lid lag - drying of the cornea / Ins ↓ blinking	eyelids	ptosis (drooping)
	hot, pulses palpable	extremities	parasthesia / numbness carpal tunnel syndrome
4	drawn, flushed, blushed	face	non-pitting oedema / puffy
	↓↓	fertility	↓↓
	↑ ↑↑ ↓ / ↑↑ ↑↑ / flatulence / diarrhoea ↑↑	GIT CHANGES - motility of GIT dysphagia cholesterol / lipids bowel movements liver function	↑ ↑↑ ↑↑ / ↑ ↓ / constipation ↓↓
5	fine thin, loss ++	hair - axillary / body	coarsening darkening loss++
6	fine thin - loss +++	hair - head	coarse dry - loss +
	↑	hearing	↑↑
	↑↑↑ ↑↑↑ ↑↑ AF / arrhythmias ↑ ↑↑	HEART/ CVS - CO RATE contractility pathology PVR	↓↓ ↓↓ ↓↓ CVD ↑ ↓↓
	↑ ↑ due to increased demands associated with goitre development	HORMONE CHANGES catecholamines EPO INS oestrogens	↓ ↑ due to reduced breakdown will decrease THs

↓ - ↓ / variable ↑ / ↑	progesterone prolactin testosterone TSH THs (T4) / iodine uptake	↓ ↑ ↑ ↓ ↑ ↑ ↓ / ↓
↑ AI Abs	Immune system	↑ AI Abs
+++++	irritability	+++
↑ ↑ ↑ ↑ ↑ ↑ NAD ↓ ↓ ↑ ↑	KIDNEY - BF GFR RAAS activity Na levels urinary concentrating ability progression to renal disease	↓ ↓ ↓ ↓ ↓ ↓ ↓ ↓ ↓ ↓ ↓
varies	libido	↓
light irregular absent	menstruation	PMT ↑
no association	menopause	*many overlapping symptoms* thyroid disease & menopause may present together even if not related
↓ ↓ proximal	muscle - mass weakness	↓ ↓ distal / ↓ cardiocontractility
soft	nails	brittle, ridged
♀ **4X > ♂**	sex bias	♀ **10X > ♂**
hot moist ↑ sweating - itching ↓ sub cut fat	skin	cold dry patches ↓ sweating non pitting oedema - myxoedema induration
insomnia ++ disturbed circadian rhythm	sleep	broken
↓ ↓	strength / muscle weakness	↓ ↓
heat intolerance - BMR ↑	temperature / BMR	cold intolerance - BMR ↓ lower body temperature
goitre discomfort / tracheal compression breathlessness	throat / thyroid / trachea	neck swelling & oedema fat deposition dry sore throat - dry cough
+++	tiredness	++++
	tongue	macroglossia
high pitch / strained	voice	deepens / coarse / ↓ volume
LOSS	weight	GAIN

Faces of thyroid disease

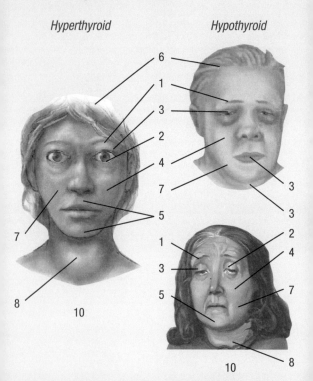

Hyperthyroid   *Hypothyroid*

Body changes with thyroid disease

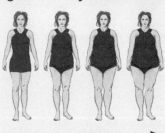

From this to this - as the thyroid function deteriorates

       © A. L. Neill

The Thyroid Hormones

T3 - the most active TH

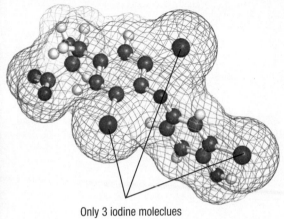

Only 3 iodine moleclues

T4 - the other TH

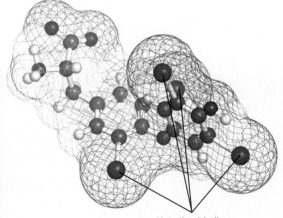

Note the 4 iodine molecules

Thyroid gland - Thyroid eye disease (TED)

Schema of eye changes in thyroid disease

Eye problems are frequently associated with thyroid disease particularly Graves' disease (an AITD), although they may develop independantly. 10% of patients do not demonstrate any overt thyroid disease but have the AI Abs to the TH receptors, which target the fibroblasts of the EOMs, causing them to become fat cells & expand, pushing the eyeball forward. A clinical schema assigns 1 point for each of the symptoms listed below. If the cumulative score > 3 the disease is active. The most serious symptoms are intense pain from ON compression (21c) & possible irreversible corneal ulceration from the exophthalmia (24). The commonest presenting age group is b/n 30-50 yo with ♀ presenting 4X more frequently than ♂. Thyroid diseases rise sharply > 60yo, particularly hypothyroiism in women.

Pain	1	Painful, oppressive feeling on or behind the globe
	2	Pain on attempted up, side or down gaze
Erythema	3	Redness of the eyelids
	4	Diffuse redness of the conjuctiva covering at least one quadrant
Odema	5	Swelling of eyelids
	6	Chemosis AKA swelling of the conjunctiva &/or watery eyes
	7	Swollen caruncle L = lateral / m = medial
	8	Increase of proptosis ≥ 2 mm causing dry irritated cornea
Impaired function	9	Decrease of eye movements in any direction ≥5°
	10	Decrease of visual acuity of ≥1 line on the Snellen chart (using a pin hole)

21 Optic N
   c = compressed

22 eye socket contents - fat & EOMs
   m =+ immune cell infiltrate, lymphocytes, monocytes & mØs

23 repair of lower lid after long standing TED

24 exophthalmia - protrusion of the eyeball from the socket

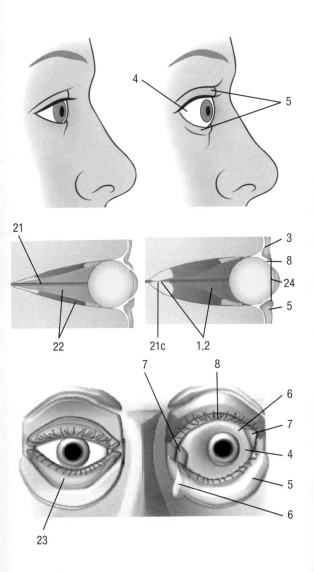

Thyroid & Pregnancy

hCG & oestrogen ↑ TH levels in the blood. hCG is made by the placenta similar to TSH & mildly stimulates the thyroid to produce more TH. Increased Oestrogen levels of pregnancy ↑ higher levels of TBG AKA thyroxine-binding globulin, a protein that transports THs in the blood, allowing for elevated levels.

Both these changes ↓ TSH levels (particularly in the 1st trimester)

THs are critical to normal development of the baby's brain & NS, particularly in the 1st 12 wks, hence hypothyroidism has more serious consequences than hyperthyroidism in pregnancy. In the first trimester, the foetus depends on the mother's supply of THs, which crosses the placenta. At 12 weeks, the baby's thyroid begins to function on its own, slowly ↑ its own TH levels. The thyroid enlarges slightly in healthy women during pregnancy, but not enough to be detected by a physical exam.

The SS of pregnant women with thyroid disease are the same as those who have primary thyroid disease, allowing for the specific differences in these patients - as indicated in the following tables.

Thyroid diseases of pregnancy	Hyperthyroidism	Hypothyroidism
prevalence	0.2% of all pregnancies	3-4% of all pregnancies
Auto Immune Disease (AID)	Graves' disease 85% of cases*	Hashimoto's disease 80%
	PPT in the pregnancy 3-8%	PPT postpartum for a yr - *predisposes the woman to permanent hypothyroidism (<30%)*
disease process	production of TSI an auto-Ab which mimics TSH elevating THs	production of anti-TBO an auto-Ab which attacks TBO preventing the formation of THs
histology changes	columnar follicular cells lymphocytic infiltration +++ in eye, skin, thyroid	fibrosis / hyperplasia ruptured follicles lymphocytic infiltration +++ oesinophilia
H changes (used as the basis of diagnosis)	TH +++ T3 in particular ↓ TSH with ↑ freeT4 presence of TSI	TH ↓ TSH +++ presence of anti-TBO
non AID based rare	hyperemesis gravidarum - severe vomiting nausea ± dehydration	
aetiology	↑ hCG which stimulates the THs production	
SS of the uncontrolled disorder		
maternal	CCF In, miscarriage placental abruption pre-eclampsia preterm delivery thyroid storm	cardiac dysfunction microcytic anaemia miscarriage placental abruption post-partum Hg pre-eclampsia (depression with PP)

neonatal / foetal	goitre (2-4X)	congenital abnormalities
	intrauterine death	hypertension
	prematurity	low birth weight
	thyrotoxicosis	poor neuropsychological
		development
		prematurity
		still birth

* note pre-existing Graves disease will improve during pregnancy & up to 2-3 mnths post-partum due to ↓IMR.

Thyroid diseases	Hyperthyroidism	Hypothyroidism
age changes	↓ age most prevalent in the reproductive years	present in the reproductive years ↑ > 60 yo in both ♂ & ♀
sex bias	♂ > ♀ up to 10X partic if AID	♀ > ♂ up to 10X partic if AID
SIGNS Eyes	severe eye changes in 30% patients diplopia exophthalmos lid lag - retraction /↓ blinking / starey appearance ophthalmopathy photophobia	periorbital puffiness ptosis
Heart	AF cardiac failure cardiomegaly ↑ first heart sound systolic murmurs tachycardia > 100 with exag. BP differences	bradycardia cardiomegaly hypotension pericardial effusion
Skin / Hair / Nails	fine, thin hair hyperhidrosis / hot to touch onycholysis - Plummer's nails	dry, yellowish hair/ skin thin brittle & sparse hair non pitting oedema pretibial myxoedema
Thyroid	goitre 2-4X variable texture ± neck swelling ± nodule ± bruit	goitre firm
other	↑ nervousness /restlessness reflexes +++++ tremor ++ weight changes	carpal tunnel syndrome deepened voice tone glossomegaly ↓ hearing paralytic ileus / ↓ bowel sounds reflexes minimal / absent
SYMPTOMS	heat intolerance ↓ concentration ↑ defecation frequency ↑ emotional lability / anxiety ↓ **fertility** muscle weakness palpitations	cold intolerance ↓ concentration constipation depression ↓ **fertility** ↑ joint stiffness ↑ muscle cramping ↑ tiredness / lethargy ↑ weight

Uterus - changes with age & H levels

1 **new born - note is larger than that of the infant**
due to the influence of the mother's Hs crossing the placenta

2 **infant about 3yo**
lowest levels of sex Hs, causes a reversion in the size of the uterus

3 **13yo girl - at puberty 1/2 above & 1/2 below the isthmus line**
under the influence of rising H levels - partic oestrogens, myometrium & mucosa thicken

4 **adult - nulliparous**

5 **adult - multiparous**
with a return to normal H levels the uterus does not retrurn to the former nulliparous size

6 **menopausal female - note there is a higher fibrous content of this organ**
↓ in ovarian Hs ↓ the mucosa & myometrium only the Hs from the adrenal cortex maintain any 2° sexual characteristics

7 **line of the isthmus & anterior peritoneal reflection note in the infant & menopausal uterus this line divides the uterus in to 2/3 cervix & 1/3 fundus reflecting similar H levels**

8 **uterine cavity of the fundus**

9 **cervix - note elongates in the pregnant uterus**

10 **os AKA entrance of the cervix**
e = external os circular in the nulliparous - slit-like
i = internal os after childbirth

11 **cervical mucous glands**
↓ after menopause as they are no longer supported by female sex Hs

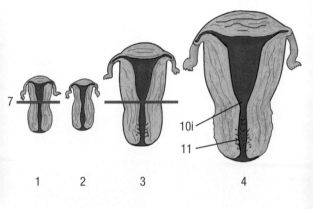

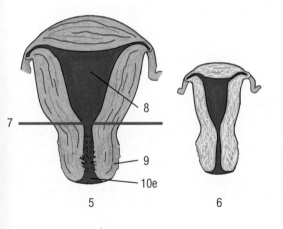

1   2   3   4

5   6

Vaginal epithelium - changes with age

	Oestrogen	Epithelium
NEW BORN	++	
1 MONTH OLD CHILD	–	
PUBERTY	present	
MATURE	+++	
MENOPAUSE post-MN	+ ➔ –	

* Doerlein bacillus AKA *Lactobacillus acidophilus* a large Gram +ve bacterium in normal vaginal secretions

© A. L. Neill

Glycogen	pH	Resident Flora
+	acid 4-5	Sterile ↓ * Doderlein's bacilli from the mother Secretion: ++++
+	alkaline >7	Coccal & ++ various flora Secretion: ++
− ➜ +	alkaline ↓ acid 7-4	Coccal + ↓ Rich bacillary
+++	acid 4-5	Lactobacillus +++ Secretion: +++
−	neutral ↓ alkaline 7-4	Varied Depending on level of circulating oestrogen Secretion: +

ANP fluid balance

LARGE FLUID INTAKE (eg. swallowing water, drowning)

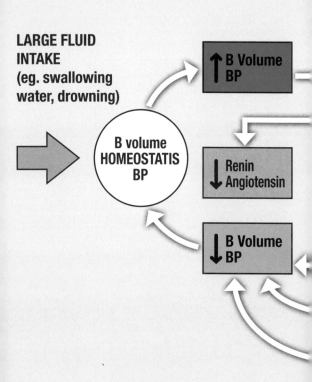

B volume HOMEOSTATIS BP

↑ B Volume BP

↓ Renin Angiotensin

↓ B Volume BP

© A. L. Neill

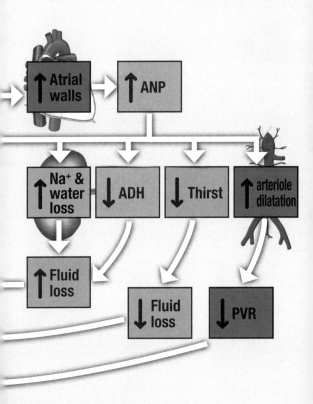

↑ **Atrial walls** → ↑ **ANP**

↑ **Na⁺ & water loss**   ↓ **ADH**   ↓ **Thirst**   ↑ **arteriole dilatation**

↑ **Fluid loss**   ↓ **Fluid loss**   ↓ **PVR**

Genitalia - external development

A   Genital tubercle - Indifferent stage
B   Genitals at 10 weeks
C   Genitals at 34 weeks
D   External genitals - fully developed

The genitals begin as an indifferent genital tubercle. Under the .
influence of oestrogen the female external genitals differentiate,
while the male genitals are formed under the influence of androgens
in particular testosterone, produced by the adrenal cortex & the
developing testes.

W/o H influence - the genitals will develop as an immature female.

	A	B	C	D
1	Glans area	Glans	Glans clitoris ♀ Glans penis ♂	Glans clitoris ♀ Glans penis ♂
2	epithelial tag	epithelial tag	epithelial tag	
3	urogenital fold	urethral fold	11 + 15 ♀ 15 ♂	11 + 15 ♀ 15 + 17 ♂
4	urogenital groove	urogenital groove		13 ♂ 13 +14 + 16 ♀
5	anal pit	anal pit		external anal opening
6	anal tubercle	anal tubercle	15	
7	lateral buttress	lateral tubercle	12 + 17 ♀ 12 ♂	
8	coronal sulcus		prepuce	prepuce
9	tail - stump (cut)			
10		labloscrotal swelling	labia majora ♀ scrotal sac ♂	labia majora ♀ scrotal sac ♂
11		urethral raphe -fused groove	penile scrotal raphe	penile scrotal raphe
12			shaft / body of the penis corpus clitoris	shaft / body of penis ♀ corpus clitoris ♂
13			urethral meatus	urethral meatus
14			labia minora ♀	labia minora - border of the vestibule ♀
15				perineal raphe
16				vaginal opening ♀
17				post. commissure ♀

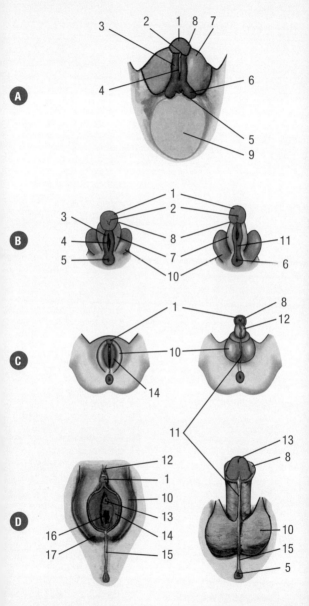

A

B

C

D

© A. L. Neill

Glucose - Utilization & Control

A Schema of Glucose metabolism in the Hepatocyte
B Schema of Glucose metabolism in the SKM & AT
C Schema of Glucose metabolism in the Brain & Nervous T

While glucose (20) can enter the hepatocyte (52c) w/o Hs or transporter systems this is not the case with AT (54) & SKM (53) which need INS (1) to allow glucose to enter their cells, while the liver needs INS to be present for glucose to leave the hepatocyte. The brain (56) needs a steady supply of glucose for its E needs or DISORIENTATION, CONVULSIONS, COMA & DEATH will result, so the level of B[glucose] needs to be tightly controlled, via Hs INS (1), CGC (3), adrenaline (2) & cortisol (4). Low B[glucose] levels stimulate adrenaline & GCG release, to breakdown glycogen (23) & release glucose, from the liver & other organs. Glucose cannot exit the liver w/o INS. Cortisol & the other glucocorticoids (4) released from the adrenal cortex also ↑ B[glucose] and is a response to stress.

The primary but not the only control of B[glucose] levels is INS, with ↑ IR the metabolic syndrome will develop. Later this may progress to DM2.

These interrelationships are demonstrated in the following diagrams, using the common code below & listed abbreviations.

Hormone Influences
0 = no hormonal or transport system needed
++ stimulated or accelerated by ...
-- inhibited or prevented by ...
  1 INS
  2 Adrenaline
  3 GCG
  4 cortisol

Substrates, Metabolites & PROCESSES
  20 Glucose
  21 G1P
  22 Uridine diphospho-glucose
  23 GLYCOGEN
  24 Pyruvic acid
  25 Lactic acid
  26 G6P
  27 F6P
  28 acetyl -CoA
     a = acetoacetyl-CoAl

     m = malonyl- CoA
     p = palmityl- CoA
  29 ammonia
  30 urea
  31 Plasma proteins
  32 tissue proteins
  33 phosphoglycerol
  34 glycerol

Structures
  50 portal vein
  51 systemic circulation
  52 liver
  c = hepatocyte
  53 SKM
  54 AT
  55 adrenal medulla
  56 brain
  57 pancreas
     a = alpha (α) cells
     b = beta (β) cells
  58 adrenal cortex

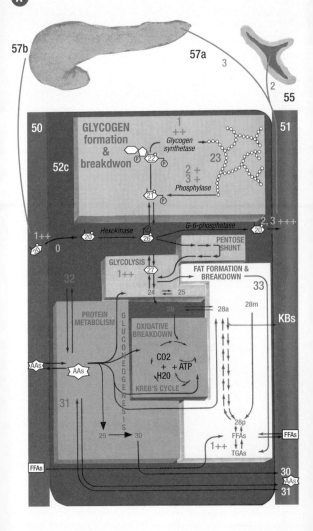

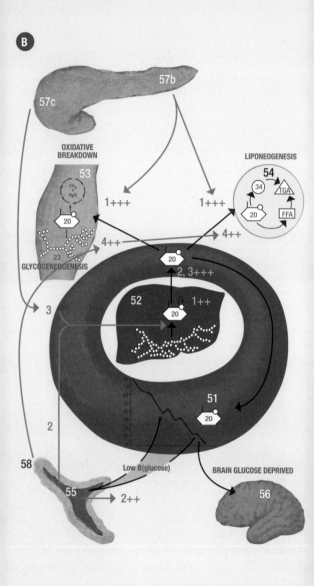

B

OXIDATIVE
BREAKDOWN

53

LIPONEOGENESIS

54

57c

57b

1+++

1+++

4++

4++

20

23

GLYCOGENEOGENESIS

34

TGA

20

FFA

20

2, 3+++

52

1++

20

3

51

20

2

58

Low B(glucose)

BRAIN GLUCOSE DEPRIVED

55

2++

56

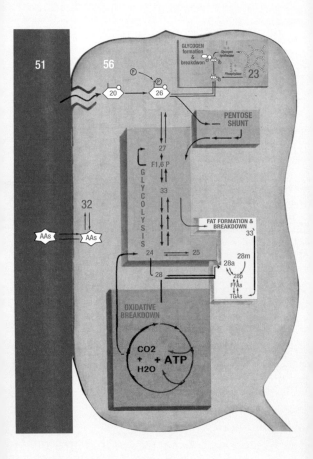

C

51 **56**

GLYCOGEN
formation
&
breakdwon

1
Glycogen
synthetase
2
Phosphylase

23

P

20 **26**

PENTOSE
SHUNT

27

F1,6 P

33

32

AAs AAs

G
L
Y
C
O
L
Y
S
I
S

**FAT FORMATION &
BREAKDOWN**

33'

24 25

28a 28m

28 28p

FFAs

TGAs

OXIDATIVE
BREAKDOWN

CO2
+ **+ ATP**
H2O

Glucose - Insulin release ß cells

Schema - cm

Increased B[glucose] causes the ß cells of the pancreas to release insulin.

1　B[glucose]
2　glucose receptor - transports glucose into the cell
3　where it is converted to pyruvate
4　& further oxidised in the mitochondria
5　forming ATP
6　this reverses K+ / ATP pump allowing
7　K+ to escape & causing
8　cm depolarization
9　opening the voltage controlled Ca++ channel
10　Ca++ acts on the
11　secretory vesicle containing
12　Insulin releasing it from the cell

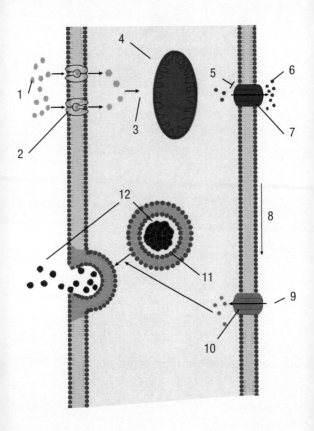

Internal gonad & sexual accessory tubular differentiation

A   sexual accessory structures indifferent stage → *birth*
B   gonad development - *F   ovary development*
                        - *M   testis development*

With the development of the gonads - the respective embryonic tubules also change - the Müllerian (paramesonephric) duct is preserved and becomes the oviduct for the ovaries & the Wolffian (mesonephric) duct which also drains the kidneys maintains its connections with the testes.

1 gonad indifferent stage
2 mesonephros
3 mesonephric duct AKA Wolffian duct
   d = degenerating
   → Oepoophoron (remnants of this duct in the broad ligament)
   → Gartner's cyst (remnants of this duct post. wall of the vagina)
4 paramesonephric duct AKA Müllerian duct
   d = degenerating
   → prostatic utricle (male equivalent of the uterus)
5 cloaca → urinary bladder
6 gonad - ovary ♀ / testis ♂
7 uterus
8 seminal vesicle
9 prostate gland
10 sex cords
   c = cortical ♀ /
   m = medullary ♂
11 oviduct -with fimbria at the end
12 vas deferens
13 epididymis
14 paradidymis
15 rete testis
16 seminiferous tubules
17 tunica albuginea of testis
18 cortex & capsule of ovary
19 primordial germ cells (spermatogonium ♂ oogonium ♀)
20 supportive nourishing cells (sustenacular cells ♂ stromal granulosa ♀)
21 ureter
22 kidney
23 vagina

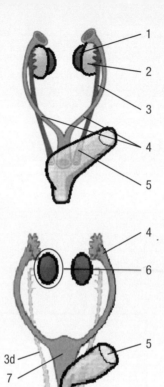

A

1
2
3
4
5

B-F

4
6
3d
7
5

B-M

6
4d
3
5
8
9

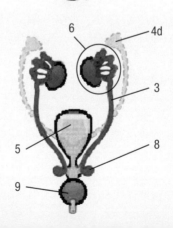

© A. L. Neill

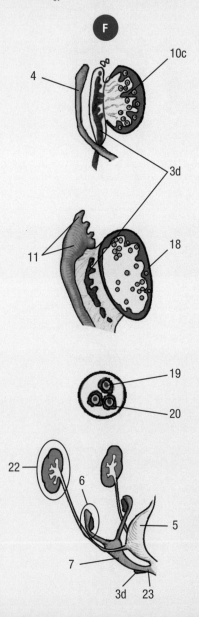

© A. L. Neill

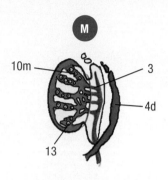

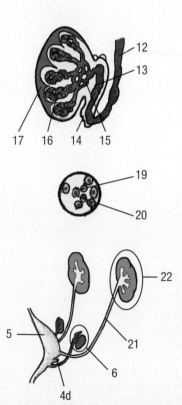

10m

3

4d

13

12

13

17   16   14   15

19

20

22

21

5

6

4d

© A. L. Neill

Menarche

Hormone changes
infancy A → childhood B → reproductive years C →
menopause D
Progesterone levels around puberty

The menarche signals the possibility of fertility, although for the first 2-3 years, the cycle may be anovulatory or have irregular ovulation. The evolution of a regular cycle is indicative of nubility - regular ovulation & fertility. The culmination of physiological & anatomical processes, combine to cause the commencement of the menses. There is no specific H signal. The average age of menarche has declined over the last century, & is now estimated to be b/n 12-14yo. It is influenced by a number of factors

These include:
- ↑ BMI - > 17% body fat (regular ovulation requires >22% body fat)
- ↑ of the GnRF pulse generation in the hypothalamic arcuate nucleus.
- ↑ oestrogen by the ovaries in response to FSH & LH (from the pituitary) which causes :
    - ↑ uterine wall & endometrium thickness, & vascularity
    - ↑ height
    - ↑ weight- specifically regional AT deposits including breast development (Thelarche)
    - ↑ pelvic widening
- induction of cyclical fluctuations of H levels via the feedback loop:
    ovary (oestrogen) → pituitary (FSH) → ovary → pituitary →
- changes of adequacy of BF to parts of the endometrium - due to H fluctuations
- necrosis of the superficial endometrial T - due to BS fluctuations
- *deciduation*, a sloughing off of the dead endometrial T into the vagina

1. LH
2. FSH
3. Oestradial
4. night- sleep
5. day -wakefulness
6. nocturnal increases of FSH & LH in puberty
7. associated morning increases in oestradial in puberty
8. maternal influence on infant H levels
9. day of expected ovulation
10. childhood - 0-9yo
11. perimenarche - 9-13yo
12. postmenarche -14-18yo

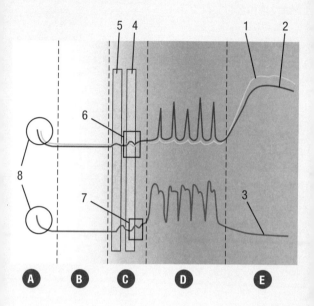

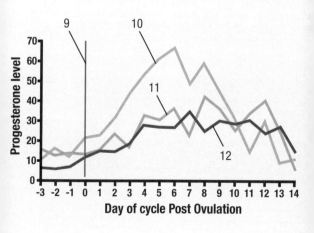

Menopause

Hormone changes - ovary output
Hormone changes - oestrogen dominance

After 35yo the ovarian output ↓ markedly- particularly the progesterone levels.

From 35yo to 50yo the progesterone decreases by 75% but the oestrogen decreases only be 35%.

Perimenopausal symptoms are present as the levels fall below half their peak levels.

1 **fertile period**
2 **symptomatic period - perimenopausal period**
3 **postmenopausal period**
4 **menopause H level**
5 **oestrogen**
6 **progesterone**

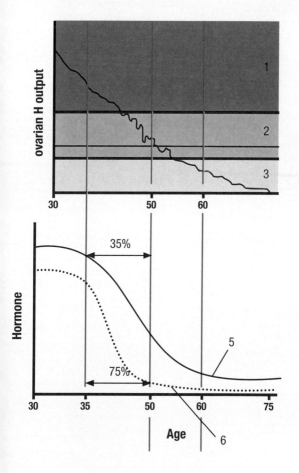

ovarian H output

1

2

3

30   50   60

Hormone

35%

75%σ

5

6

30   35   50   60   75

Age

© A. L. Neill

Menopause

Hormone changes - before & after
Hormone patterns 6 months   - *premenopause*   A
                                    - *perimenopause*   B
                                    - *postmenopause*   C

At the menopause the FSH & LH levels rise to > 4X that in the fertile years unrestrained by the oestrogen negative feedback loop, as the ovary H output diminishes.

1   **Oestradiol**
2   **Oestrogens**
3   **FSH**
4   **LH**
5   **menopause**
6   **Progesterone**

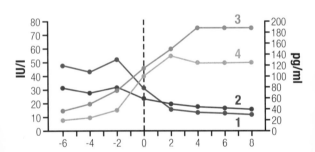

     © A. L. Neill

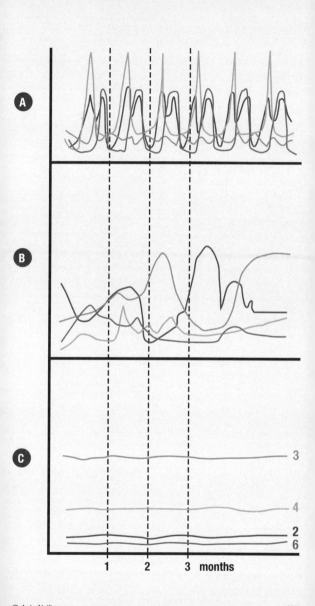

Menopause - changes to bone

With the reduction oestradiol & oestrogen production, osteoblasts stop producing OPG.

OPG binds to RANKL mopping it up & stopping it from binding to the surface bound RANK receptor on bone cells & osteoclasts. The RANKL/RANK complex ↑ osteoclast formation & activation.

Osteoclasts resorb bone. This may lead to osteoporosis.

1 **OPG produced by osteoblasts**
2 **RANKL**
3 **OPG/RANKL complex**
4 **osteoblast**
5 **RANK - surface receptor**
6 **RANKL/RANK complex**
7 **osteoclast - inactive**
8 **bone**
9 **osteoclast activated**
10 **bone resorption**

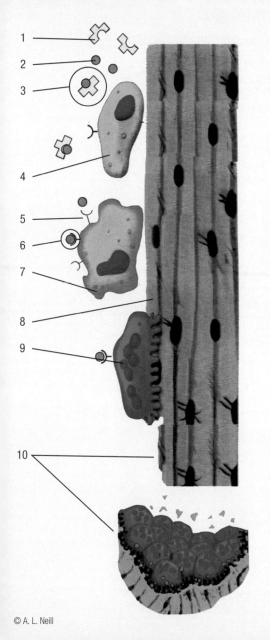

1
2
3
4
5
6
7
8
9
10

© A. L. Neill

Menopause - organ pathophysiology overview

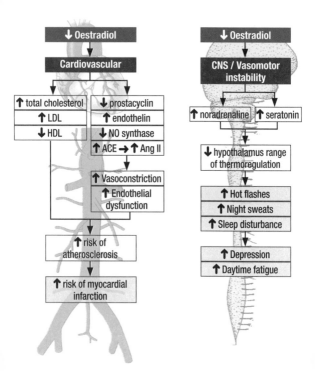

↓ Oestradiol

Cardiovascular

↑ total cholesterol
↑ LDL
↓ HDL

↓ prostacyclin
↑ endothelin
↓ NO synthase
↑ ACE → ↑ Ang II

↑ Vasoconstriction
↑ Endothelial dysfunction

↑ risk of atherosclerosis

↑ risk of myocardial infarction

↓ Oestradiol

CNS / Vasomotor instability

↑ noradrenaline   ↑ seratonin

↓ hypothalamus range of thermoregulation

↑ Hot flashes
↑ Night sweats
↑ Sleep disturbance

↑ Depression
↑ Daytime fatigue

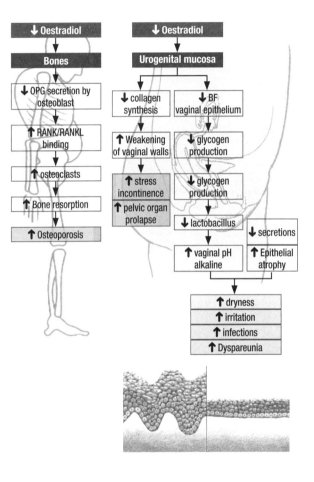

↓ Oestradiol

Bones

↓ OPG secretion by osteoblast

↑ RANK/RANKL binding

↑ osteoclasts

↑ Bone resorption

↑ Osteoporosis

↓ Oestradiol

Urogenital mucosa

↓ collagen synthesis

↑ Weakening of vaginal walls

↑ stress incontinence
↑ pelvic organ prolapse

↓ BF vaginal epithelium

↓ glycogen production

↓ glycogen production

↓ lactobacillus

↑ vaginal pH alkaline

↓ secretions

↑ Epithelial atrophy

↑ dryness
↑ irritation
↑ infections
↑ Dyspareunia

© A. L. Neill

Menstral Cycle - *feedback loops*

Hypothalamic control of menstruation

- ■ GnRH stimulates FSH
- ■ FSH -stimulates follicle development
- ▨ LH -stimulates oestradial production
- ■ Oestrogen / Oestradial stimulates endometrial growth inhibits FSH & GnRH
- ▨ Inhibin inhibits FSH

— inhibitory pathways

— stimulatory pathways

1 **Hypothalamus**
2 **Pituitary -**
     a = anterior / p = posterior
3 **Follicle**
4 **Ovary**
5 **Endometrium**

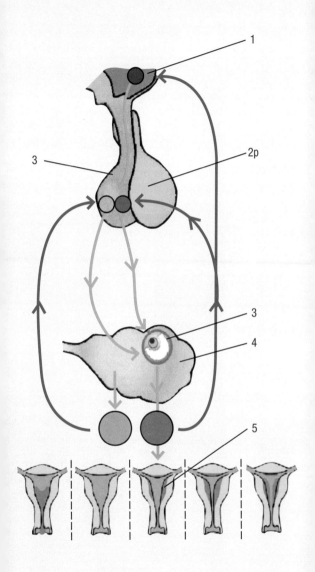

Menstrual Cycle & Exercise Training

Menstrual Week	1		2
Menstrual Days	1 to 5	6 to 8	9 to 12
Phase	Early Follicular (Menses)	Mid Follicular	Late Follicular
Hormone Levels	T, O & P ↓	O ↗ P ↘ GH ↑	O ↑ P ↓
Physiological & Psychological changes	↑ mood change ↑ irritability ↑ stress ↓ reaction times ↓ immune system	↑ glycogen storage & tissue uptake	↑ glycogen, electrolyte, fat, protein stores
Ideal Training	↑ Strength & Power training ↓ Complex Precision training	↑ Light exercise ↓ Weight bearing	↑ Strength & Power training ↑ Complexity
Intensity	↓ Light	→	↗ Increasing

Testosterone (T) - Oestrogen (O) - Progesterone (P) - Growth Hormone (GH)

2	3	4	
13 to 14	15 to 20	21 to 24	25 to 31
Ovulation	Early Luteal	Mid Luteal	Late Luteal
O ↑ T ↑	O → P ↗	O → P ↑	T, O & P ↓
↑ breast size ↑ vaginal mucus viscosity ↑ body temp +/- abdominal pain / bloating	↑ total E ↑ fat intake ↑ lipolysis ↑ water & electrolyte retention ↓ B[lactate]	↑ protein breakdown ↑ glycogen, fat, protein stores ↑ water & electrolyte retention ↓ muscular endurance	↑ mood changes ↑ irritability ↑ stress ↓ reaction times ↓ immune system
↑ Strength & Power training ↑ Complexity		↑ Light exercise ↑ Endurance ↓ Weight bearing	↑ Strength & Power training ↓ Complex Precision training
↑ Maximum	↘ Decreasing	→	↓ Light

Menstruation
Hormone levels

Schema

The hypothalamus releases GnRF = GONADOTROPIN RELEASING FACTOR (i.e. a substance which allows for the secretion secondary substances which will cause the growth of follicles in the ovary) = 1

The anterior pituitary gland releases FSH = FOLLICLE STIMULATING HORMONE (i.e. a substance which stimulates the growth of follicles in the ovary) = 2

The anterior pituitary gland releases LH = LUTEINIZING HORMONE (i.e. a substance which stimulates the growth of the follicle in the ovary. It also causes ovulation - the release of an ovum from a mature follicle when it surges in the middle of the menstral cycle) = 3 *under the influence of the peak OE level.*

The ovarian follicle (FL) as it grows produces OE = OESTROGEN in increasing amounts, until ovulation = 4

The ovarian corpus luteum (CL) forms from the follicle after the release of the ovum. It continues to produce OE (4) at lower levels & starts to produce PR = PROGESTERONE = 5

The uterine wall grows thicker & more vascular under the influence of OE & PR

The hypothalamus stops producing GnRF (1) under the influence of OE & PR.

So the anterior pituitary stops producing FSH

The CL stops growing and stops producing OE & PR.

The uterine wall is no longer stimulated to grow and is shed.

The cycle begins again.

Day 1 is generally referred to as the beginning of the cycle, during the menstral or bleeding period.

Day 14 is generally the day of ovulation - mid cycle.

Most cycles are b/n 22 to 35 days, although there is considerable variation.

The cycle is divided into the FOLLICULAR PHASE (before ovulation) = F & the LUTEAL PHASE (after ovulation) = L. At ovulation (O) the egg/ovum is released and travels along the ovarian tubes to towards the uterus where it is usually shed.

1 **GnRF**
2 **FSH**
3 **LH**
4 **Oestrogen (OE)**
5 **Progesterone (PR)**

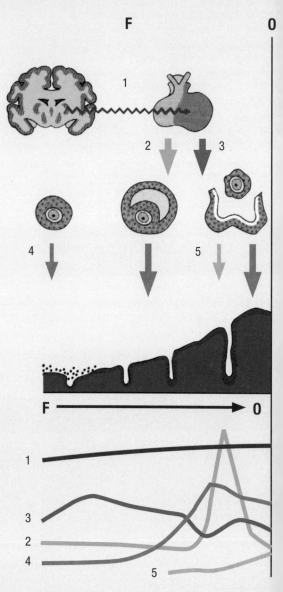

© A. L. Neill

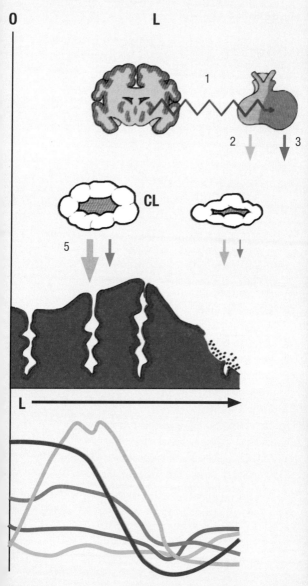

O L

1

2 3

CL

5

L

Ovulation *Schema*

Secondary Follicle - pre-ovulation
Tertiary Follicle - Ovulation

■ FSH - stimulates the swelling & breakaway of cumulus orpheus
   activates plasminogen

■ PGs - causing lysis of germinal epithelium, which releases
   lysozymes contraction of the SM - ↑ P in the follicle

■ Plasmin activator

■ LH - activates PGs
      stimulates meiosis in the oocyte
      starts luteinization of the theca & granulosa

■ plasminogen → plasmin (active form)

■ lysozymes which dissolves the stigma

1 **primary oocyte - stopped at dictyotene
   (METAPHASE I of meiosis)**
2 **secondary oocyte + 1st polar body - meiosis has
   resumed**
3 **germinal epithelium - surface of the ovary**
4 **theca interna cellular layer**
5 **granulosa**
6 **follicular liquor**
7 **BM of the follicle**
8 **BM of the germinal epithelium**
9 **stigma - in place - dissolves at ovulation**
10 **BM - Zona Pellucida of the oocyte**
11 **Cumulus Orpheus - swollen at ovulation**

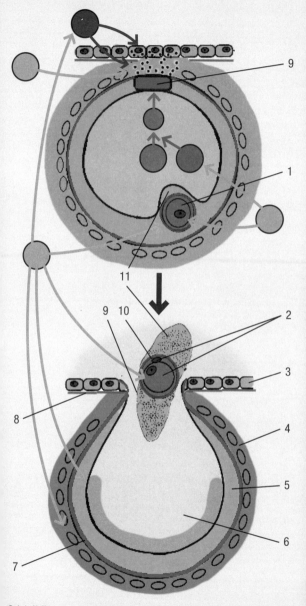

© A. L. Neill

Ovulation *Hormone levels*

BT - Body Temperature
AP - Anterior Pituitary H levels
OH - Ovarian H levels
0 - Ovulation - period of greatest fertility

A - Menstral phase - shedding of the endometrial top 2/3
B - Proliferative phase - growth of the endometrium
C - Secretory phase - formation of the CL

■ FSH

■ Progesterone

■ LH

■ Oestrogen / Oestradial

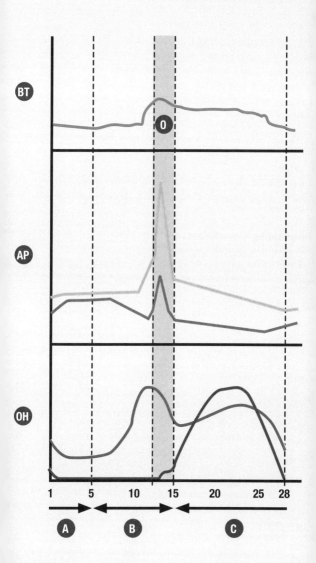

© A. L. Neill

Salt & Water homeostasis

A Water / Volume changes (Wd - water deficit, We - water excess)
B Salt concentration changes (Sd - salt deficit, Se - salt excess)

When water levels are altered the osmolarity & pressure of the CVS is altered, triggering baroreceptors and osmoreceptors to send afferent signals to the Hypothalamus. With ↑ osmolarity RF from the hypothalamus are sent to the post. pituitary releasing ADH. ADH ↑ & conserves water ↓ urine output in the kidneys.

With ↑ in volume of water the atrium of the heart releases ANF, which reacts on the Hypothalamus to ↓ RF & ↓ ADH & ↑ urine output from the kidneys.

With ↑ in salt - the plasma volume is also increased triggering ANF release & ↓ ADH. With ↓ in salt - & plasma volume ↓ triggering renin release from the afferent arteriole granular cells of the renal juxtaglomerular apparatus. **Renin AKA Angiotensinogenase** activates Angiotensinogen (circulating) to Angiotensin I - active vasoconstrictor. Circulating Angiotensin 1 is converted to Angiotensin II - most active vasoconstrictor in the lungs by endothelial bound **Angiotensin Converting Enzyme (ACE)** Angiotensin II causes Aldosterone ↑ which affects the DCT of the kidneys to conserve sodium. Angiotensin II also causes CNS to ↑ water intake by stimulating the thirst centre of the hypothalamus, & ↑ RFs & ↑ ADH.

0 = osmolarity	d = decrease	i = increase
P = Blood Pressure	d = decrease	i = increase
S = salt / sodium	d = decrease	i = increase
U = urine	d = decrease	i = increase
V = volume of fluids in the body	d = decrease	i = increase
W = water	d = decrease	i = increase

A = angiotensin
  g = proenzyme - angioteninogen
  1 = angiotensin 1, Lung, site of conversion 1 - 2 (active form)
  2 = angiotensin 2
  i = increase

  1   **thirst centre of hypothalamus**
  2   **post. pituitary site of ADH release**
  3   **kidney**
  4   **juxtaglomerular apparatus - site of renin release**
  5   **adrenal cortex site of aldosterone release**
  6   **atria of the heart - site of ANF release**

A

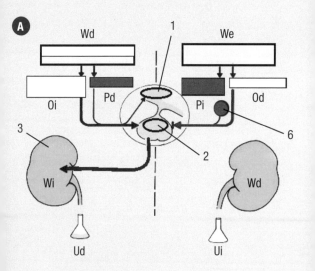

Wd   1   We

Oi   Pd   Pi   Od

3

Wi

Wd

Ud   Ui

2

6

B

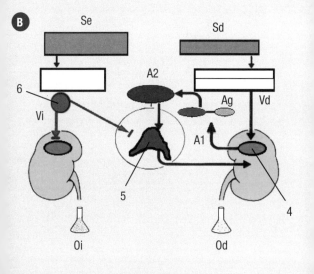

Se   Sd

6

A2

Ag

Vi   Vd

A1

5

4

Oi   Od

Stress Response

Schema of hypothalamic adrenal axis for long & short term stress

A   short term stress mediated by SymNS

B   long term stress mediated by Anterior Pituitary

	SHORT TERM RESPONSE (s)	**LONG TERMS RESPONSE (L)**
1	Ns in the hypothalamus	neurosecretory cells in the hypothalamus secreting RFs
2	long post-ganglionic fibres of the Sym NS - transmitter noradrenaline	BV plexus from the hypothalamus carrying RFs to the ant pituitary which releases ACTH
3	**secretions of noradrenaline**	**secretions of glucocorticoids** switching from glucose to FAT & PROTEIN metabolism
4	**secretions of adrenaline**	**secretions of mineralocorticoids** NA & WATER RETENTION
5	from the adrenal medulla (10% of adrenal wgt - from the neuroectoderm)	from the adrenal cortex (90% of the adrenal wgt - from mesodermal mesoderm)
effects	↑ B[glucose], ↑ HR ↑ BP B directed to the SKM	↓ IfR & IR, ↑ BP

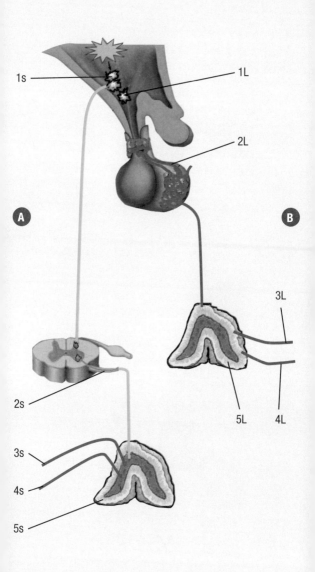

1s

1L

2L

A

B

2s

3L

5L

4L

3s

4s

5s

© A. L. Neill

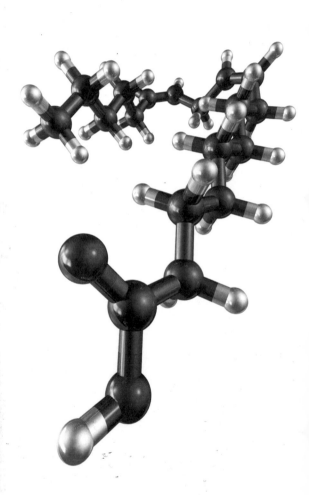

© A. L. Neill